WILD DRUGS

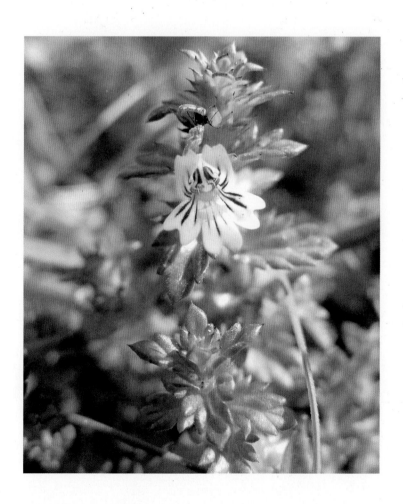

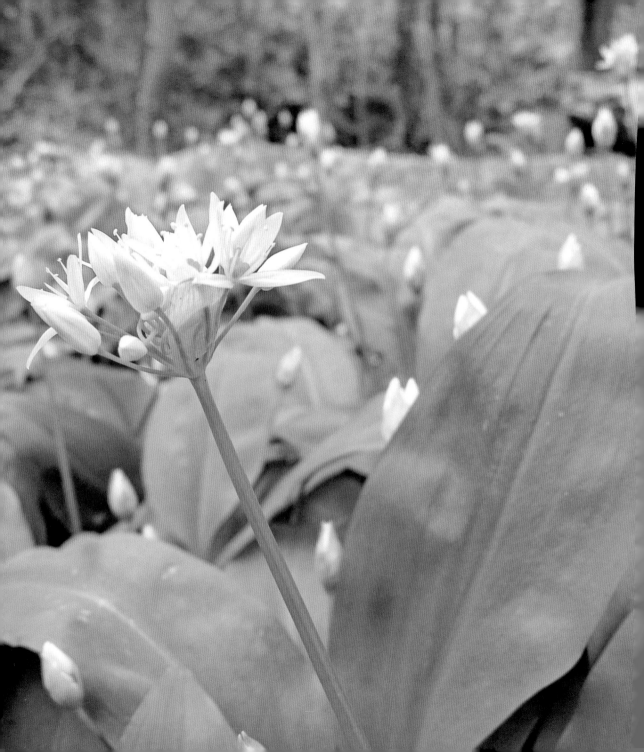

WILD DRUGS

a forager's guide to healing plants

Zoë Hawes

RGN Dip. Phyt. MNIMH

An Hachette UK Company
www.hachette.co.uk

First published in Great Britain in 2010 by
Gaia, a division of Octopus Publishing Group Ltd
Endeavour House
189 Shaftesbury Avenue
London
WC2H 8JG
www.octopusbooks.co.uk

ISBN 978-1-85675-310-4

A CIP catalogue record for this book is available
from the British Library

Printed and bound in China

10 9 8 7 6 5 4 3 2 1

Disclaimer

The views expressed in the book are those
of the Author and are not those held by the
Publisher and you are urged to consult a
relevant and qualified specialist for
individual advice in particular situations.

Many wild plants are poisonous, even
fatally poisonous. Foragers should always
identify by all indicators before using
plants obtained from the wild. Different
plants might look very similar to the
untrained eye. If you do collect wild plants
to use at home make sure that all of the
identification checks for each species are
carried out in detail to avoid poisonous
look-alikes. If in any doubt do not use the
wild plant. Beginners should have their
own identifications checked by an expert
in the field.

The Publisher and Author do not have any
intention of providing specific medical
advice and the content of this book should
not be used as a basis for diagnosis or
choice of treatment, but rather as a source
of information. All content contained in
this book is provided for this purpose only
and nothing in this book is intended to be
a substitute for professional medical
advice, care diagnosis or treatment.

The Publisher is not responsible or liable
for any diagnosis made by a reader based
on the information in this book and does
not warrant or guarantee the accuracy or
completeness of the advice in this book.
The reader's use of the content, for
whatever purpose, is at their own risk.

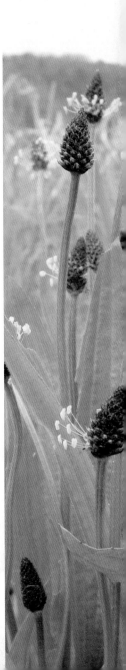

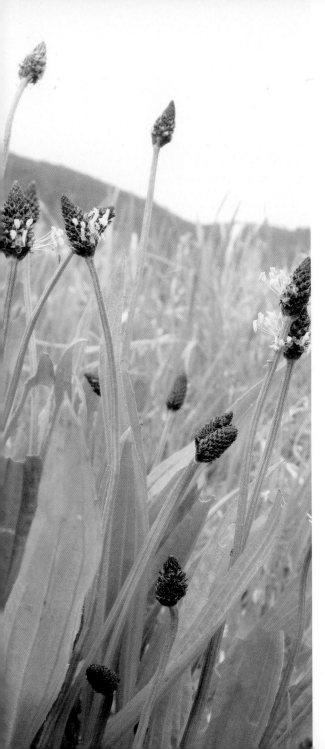

Contents

Introduction to nature's medicines

This book is a complete guide to discovering and learning about the wonderful world of healing plants that grow prolifically all around us. Many weeds that invade our parks and gardens have potent healing properties that can be safely used at home to treat a whole range of minor and common ailments. They can also be gathered for free!

This book will enable you to experience the joy of finding these plants in your immediate surroundings and the special feeling that gathering and preparing them gives. It will also instruct you on what to take, and how to take it, in order to heal yourself and your family, using what nature has provided.

Give it time

Herbs are not an instant, miracle cure, but they do have profound, tangible effects and will always help if used correctly and given time to do so. They do not bring about miracle cures because they help the body to heal itself, and healing always takes time. To succumb to illness, the body must be weakened in some way; through the gentle, supportive action of herbs, it will eventually return to a healthy equilibrium, and is often stronger than before.

What will herbs treat?

With a little knowledge and consistent application, you can safely and successfully treat minor ailments with herbs at home. Herbs can shorten the duration and severity of most common ailments, stop complications such as secondary infections and prevent them from becoming a chronic problem. Chronic problems with long-term treatment can be significantly eased by herbal medicine. It is also possible (at best) to halt the onset of an acute illness if the first signs are acted on quickly enough.

How to use this book

First, read about the legal and safety issues regarding harvesting (see pages 14–15) to ensure that you do not inadvertently harvest plants unsustainably or illegally. 'How to Forage' (see pages 10–23) includes a basic section on botany to aid identification, and includes leaf and flower shapes, plant structure and family descriptions. It also gives advice on how to harvest each individual part of the plant. 'Using Medicinal Plants' (see pages 24–35) then gives you all the information you need on how to process, store and prepare the plants for medicinal use.

The plant description chapters contain detailed profiles of 54 plants, which have been grouped by habitat: Woodland Plants (see pages 36–61), Riverside Plants (see pages 62–81), Grassland Plants (see pages

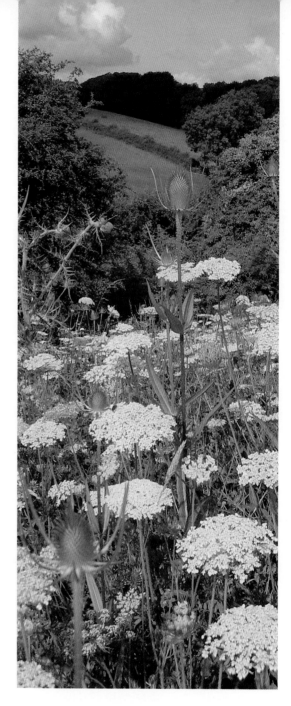

82–119), Waste Ground Plants (see pages 120–163), Hedgerow Plants (see pages 164–189) and Garden Visitors (see pages 190–209). Each plant listing gives details on the plant's folklore, its historical and modern uses, how to identify it, when and where to look for it, what to harvest, what it is good for and how to use it. There is a handy 'Forager's checklist' that you can use as a quick reference guide. Both scientific and common names are provided, and sometimes their sources, as these are often a useful memory aid regarding the plant's medicinal properties. It is a good idea to learn all about each plant and decide whether you need it in your home remedy cabinet. To get started quickly, look at the First Aid Kit (see pages 248–249), which lists the top ten healing plants for common ailments.

You can use the book in a number of different ways, depending on your needs. If you suffer with a recurrent ailment, refer to the 'Remedies for Common Ailments' chapter (see pages 210–247) to gain a deeper understanding of the problem and identify which herbs may help. Then read about them in their appropriate chapter and find out where they grow. Discover how to gather, prepare and store them so you have them to hand when you need them, and learn how to use the herb to treat yourself. Finally, refer to 'Using Medicinal Plants' (see pages 24–35) for further information on uses and doses.

Alternatively, if you are planning a walk in a wood, for example, refer to the 'Woodland Plants' chapter (see pages 36–61) and discover which plants grow there that you might wish to gather.

Wild flower meadows at the height of their growth provide rich sources of medicinal plants.

Introduction to nature's medicines

History of medicinal plants

Herbal medicine is a natural and ancient form of medicine. Primitive humans probably had an innate ability to sense which plants had healing properties, an ability still witnessed in animals today. This knowledge has been passed down through the generations for thousands of years.

The beginnings of herbalism

The earliest evidence of plant use as medicine was in a grave of a Neanderthal man, in Iraq, dating from 60,000 years ago. Plant pollens around the body were found to be from plants that are still used medicinally today. The first written record is from China (2800 BC) and includes 366 medicinal plants. Records are also found on papyrus and clay tablets from India, Egypt and Persia (now Iran). These records show us that during those times people were using many of the same plants that are still used for healing the body today, and that they had an in-depth knowledge of their properties and actions.

Hippocrates (c. 460–377 BC), the famous Greek physician who is known as the 'Father of Medicine', introduced 'holism' by writing about the treatment of the whole person, physically, mentally and spiritually. He wrote about the natural harmony in the healthy person and that in 'dis-ease' there is an upset in this balance. The role of the physician was to help the patient to help him or herself. He worked on the principles of the four humours – blood, bile, phlegm and choler – and the four elements – earth, air, fire and water. Similar elemental systems are found in Indian Ayurvedic and Chinese traditional theories of medicine.

Another Greek physician, Dioscorides (c. AD 40–90), wrote De Materia Medica, recording all his knowledge on the medicinal plants being used at that time. Galen (c. AD 129–200), another Greek physician, studied at the Alexandrian School, which combined Greek, Egyptian and Persian wisdom. He wrote a herbal, expanding on Hippocrates' ideas, that became the basis for medical learning throughout the Roman world, and continued in use until medieval times. It was brought to Britain by the Romans, where it was combined with the traditional knowledge of the Druids (who never wrote anything down).

Medieval herbalism

Throughout the Dark Ages (c. AD 300–800), Christian Rome suppressed much of this knowledge in Europe. It did not re-emerge until the Crusaders brought back plant lore derived from Arab traditions that had continued to evolve, one of the best known Arab herbalists being Avicenna. The medieval monasteries continued this learning about healing, reproducing many ancient herbals and establishing medicinal gardens. Traditional healers continued to practise outside the monasteries; the physicians of Myddfai, and one of their documents, the Leech Book of Bald (written c. AD 900), are famous examples of this.

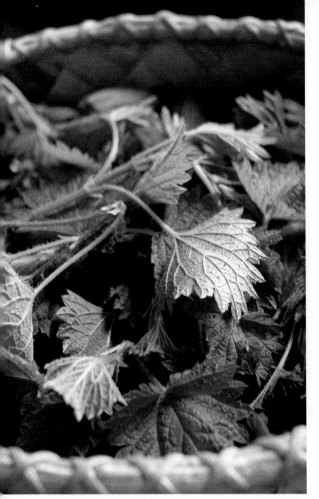

Traditional methods of harvesting medicinal plants remain appropriate and continue today.

Famous herbals

The 16th and 17th centuries saw the writing of many herbals, including *The Herbal* (1597) by John Gerard, *A New Herball* (in three parts from 1551 to 1568) by William Turner, and Nicholas Culpeper's *The English Physitian* (1652). Culpeper was a noted apothecary who translated the physicians' Latin pharmacopoeia into English so that other apothecaries could study it and treat poor patients who could not afford the doctors' fees. Culpeper used astrology in his approach, assigning astrological signs to herbs and diseases.

Modern times

In the 19th century, Samuel Thompson developed a system of frontier medicine in America from the traditional medicine used by Native Americans. It was introduced to England and many indigenous American herbs gained popularity from that. Many modern medicines began to be created using plant medicines, and these evolved until current times; now they are mostly chemically synthesized and given in standard doses. The National Institute of Medical Herbalists was established in 1864 and is the oldest existing regulating body of herbalists.

Medical herbalists continue to be trained and practise throughout the UK today, using the traditional knowledge gathered throughout history. They also benefit from modern science shedding light on the way that plants work in the body, and from their experience of treating people and observing the effects of their botanical medicines.

The Doctrine of Signatures

The 'Doctrine of Signatures' was first written about in a herbal by Paracelsus (1493–1541) in the 16th century, and was probably developed from older ideas. It outlined his belief that God gave a sign within the healing plants to indicate their medicinal properties. A good example is the tubers of pilewort that resemble piles on the bottom of the plant!

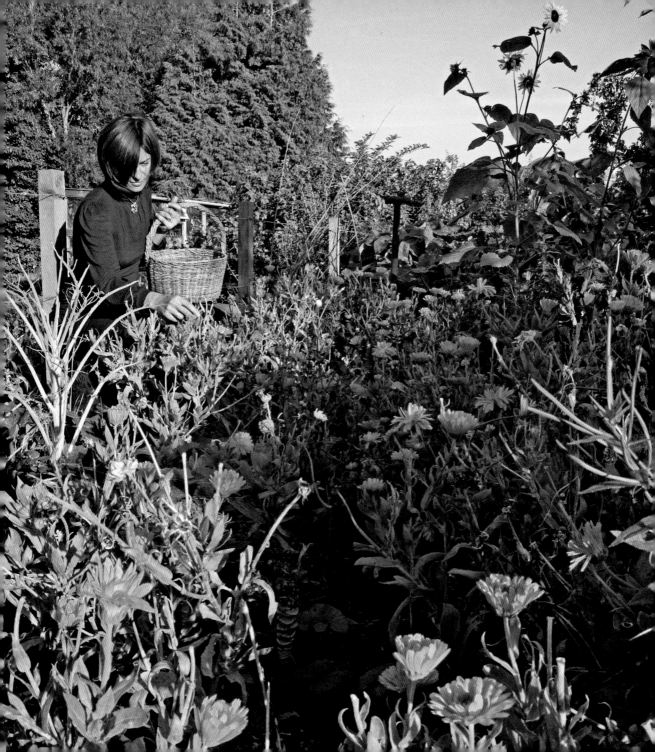

HOW TO FORAGE

Collecting enough medicinal plants to meet all your needs for a year's worth of medicine is a time-consuming pastime but one that has its own special healing properties. Get to know the plants that grow in your locality and discover all of their purposes. Be aware of all your senses and slow your pace to that of the natural environment, to enjoy the soothing effect it has on your spirit.

Harvesting plants

Here are some general rules that apply to the various plant parts, but some herbs will have special requirements that are mentioned in their particular entry.

General guidelines

- Handle plants gently to avoid bruising, which will affect constituents.
- Collect on a dry day, after the dew has dried but before the heat of the sun gets too hot and evaporates any volatile oils.
- Harvest at the right time of year for the part of the plant you want.
- Harvest away from obvious sources of pollution.
- Do not harvest diseased or damaged plants.
- Do not over-harvest and gather more than can be feasibly prepared in one go (see pages 14–15).

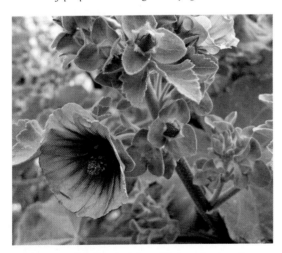

When you are foraging, look for wild plants that are vibrant, healthy and full of energy.

Whole plants and plant parts

Cut the main stem (or stems) at ground level when the plant is about to flower, and strip off any dirty or insect-infested leaves. With perennials, only gather a third of the plant's growth to allow seed to form and to avoid exhausting the roots. Leave some annuals to go to seed.

Roots

Harvest roots in early spring just as the plant begins to grow, or in late autumn when the tops have died down. Harvest biennials in autumn of the first year, or early spring before they flower. For widespread roots, dig in a broad circle around the base of the plant and lift out a large lump of earth containing the roots. Knock off the earth to reveal the roots. Taproots often grow very deep. Find the base of the plant and excavate carefully around it until the root top is exposed. Then dig away in a wider circle, following the root down as far as possible. Use a stick to loosen compacted earth and try to remove the entire root.

Leaves

Either pluck leaves off the stem with your fingers or, if the leaf stalks are tough, cut them with a sharp knife to avoid damaging the stem. This way, the stem may put forward new leaves that can be harvested again in a few weeks.

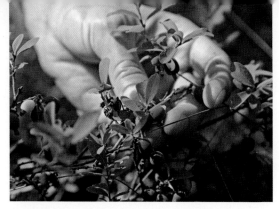

Harvesting berries by hand is slow but rewarding work. Remember to harvest them just before they ripen.

Flowers

Pick flowers when most of them are at their peak. Some flowers can be harvested continuously over a number of days or weeks. If they grow on a many-branching stem, like elderflowers, cut the whole stem and snip the flowers off individually at home. Ensure you cut the flower close to its base, excluding as much stem as possible.

Seeds

When the seedhead is almost ready to drop its seeds, take a paper bag and tie it over the seedhead, securing it to the stem. It may be left for a few days if the weather is fine. Alternatively, cut the stem and hang it upside down to allow the seeds to drop off naturally over a few days. You can then strip any remaining ones into the bag.

Berries

Pick berries when they are just about to ripen. If they are growing on a many-stemmed stalk, like elderberries, cut off the whole stalk and strip the berries off with a fork at home. Pick single berries individually by hand (wear rubber gloves if you wish to avoid staining your fingers).

Bark

Harvest bark in the spring when it peels away easily. Never strip the bark from the main trunk or in a complete circle round a branch, as the tree beyond that point will die. Look for fallen branches after a storm to harvest bark from. Alternatively, cut off a 3–5-year-old branch with a sharp pruning saw. To remove the bark, using a sharp knife score round the circumference in two places about 20 cm (8 in) apart, then score longitudinally between them. Slip the point of the knife between the bark and the core of the wood and prise back the bark along its length, then peel off in a sheet.

Sap

Sap exudes from the stems of plants when they are broken. Break a plant stem and apply it directly to the skin as required. It cannot easily be collected and stored.

Equipment you will need

* **Gardening gloves – thorn- and prickle-proof**
* **Rubber gloves**
* **Secateurs – sharp and with a safety catch**
* **Pruning saw – foldable and with a lockable blade**
* **Penknife – foldable and with a lockable blade (only needs a small, sharp blade)**
* **Trowel**
* **Basket – preferably with a large handle and finely woven so that it can hang off your arm, leaving both hands free**
* **Paper bags**

Foraging safely and legally

You must always be aware of the legal and sustainability issues when harvesting plants from the wild. There are no endangered or protected plants in this book – most of the plants described are prolific weeds that rapidly regenerate.

Sustainable harvesting guidelines

- Be aware of which plants easily and rapidly regenerate and which do not; then you can safely harvest more of the former without damaging their numbers.
- Harvest from areas that are well known to you, and return every year to see if you are having an impact on the plant population.
- Only gather up to a third of a healthy group of the same plant; more than this and you risk weakening the population.

- Only harvest from healthy, well-stocked areas. If you find a plant you would like to harvest, but it is not abundant, it is best to leave it and hope it flourishes in future years.
- Have an awareness of the impact that your presence and harvesting has on the whole environment of the area, including insect, bird and mammal life.
- Ensure that you propagate plants by scattering seed or by replanting a portion of rootstock and crown, and leave mature, well-established plants to produce future generations.
- Try to leave no impression of your harvest, by spreading your picking evenly throughout the plant growth and by replacing earth and turf from any holes you dig.
- Never harvest more than you need and can use in one go. Plants left for more than a few hours without being prepared properly lose potency.

Pollution

Harvest away from obvious pollutants, such as on busy roadsides or verges where dogs may have been, and be aware that arable and crop fields are likely to have been sprayed. If you are asking permission from farmers or land owners to harvest on their land, also ask them if, when and where they spray. Chemical

Plant populations are directly linked to the health of an ecosystem of any area, including insects and animals.

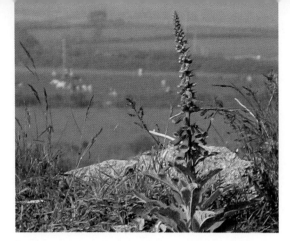

Foxglove is a common plant with toxic properties whose young leaves may be easily mistaken for medicinal plants.

Be especially careful when harvesting plants of the Umbelliferae family, as it contains some of the most poisonous European plants, including hemlock (*Conium maculatum*) and hemlock water dropwort (*Oenanthe crocata*). Other common poisonous plants in Europe are:

- Cuckoo pint (*Arum maculatum*)
- Foxglove (*Digitalis purpurea*)
- Bluebell (*Hyacinthoides non-scripta*)
- Holly (*Ilex* spp.)
- Laurel (*Prunus laurocerasus*)
- Ragwort (*Senecio jacobea*)
- Woody nightshade (*Solanum dulcamara*)

herbicides and pesticides leave their residues in the soil for many years and fertilizers give plants high levels of nitrates.

Safety

Although standard doses do apply for many plants, there are those that require much smaller doses and which will have purgative or toxic effects if taken in standard doses or for long periods. Those plants that only require smaller doses are specified in each individual herbal entry.

Poisonous plants

It is imperative to be entirely certain of what you are harvesting. If you are in any doubt about a plant, do not gather it or use it. It is important to be familiar with poisonous herbs, especially those in your area, to avoid confusion. Unwanted toxic effects from plants include skin irritation, vomiting and diarrhoea, hallucinations and life-threatening organ damage. If adverse symptoms are experienced, seek emergency medical assistance. If possible, keep a sample of the plant, fresh or dried, to assist in identification.

Obey the law

✽ It is illegal to pick or uproot any endangered plant or flower (a list of protected and endangered plants is contained in the Wildlife and Countryside Act; see www.jncc.gov.uk).

✽ It is illegal to harvest plants on private property unless you have permission from the land owner.

✽ It is illegal to harvest plants from nature reserves or Sites of Special Scientific Interest (SSSIs).

✽ On public land (local authority) and in national parks, you must obtain the proper permits and permissions from the appropriate authorities of the park you wish to visit (see the website www.nationalparks.gov.uk or your local wildlife trust).

Foraging safely and legally

How to identify plants

There are many similar-looking plants, and it is vitally important that you can identify the right one for medicinal purposes. The use of some specialized terms is unavoidable; this section will explain these for you.

Basic botany

Basic plant structures

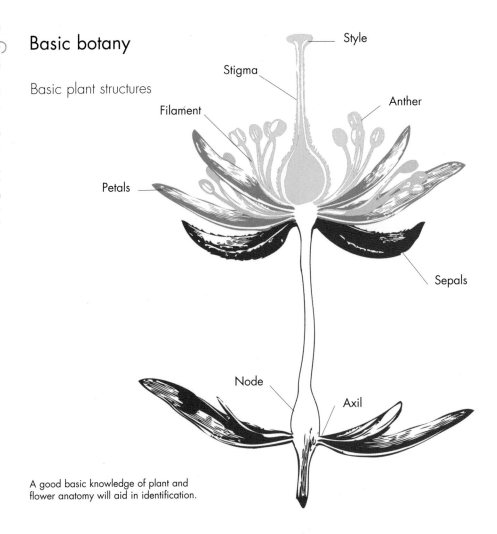

Style

Stigma

Anther

Filament

Petals

Sepals

Node

Axil

A good basic knowledge of plant and flower anatomy will aid in identification.

Leaf shapes

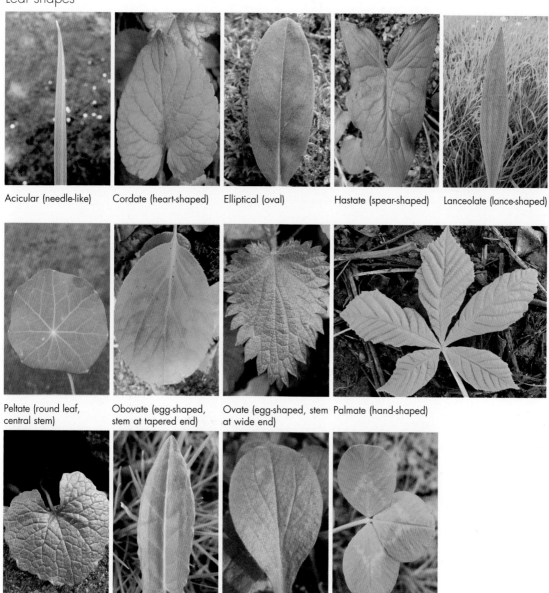

Acicular (needle-like)

Cordate (heart-shaped)

Elliptical (oval)

Hastate (spear-shaped)

Lanceolate (lance-shaped)

Peltate (round leaf, central stem)

Obovate (egg-shaped, stem at tapered end)

Ovate (egg-shaped, stem at wide end)

Palmate (hand-shaped)

Reniform (kidney-shaped)

Sagittate (arrow-shaped)

Spatulate (spoon-shaped)

Trifoliate (three leaflets)

How to identify plants

How to forage

Stem shapes

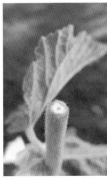 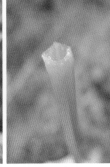 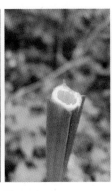 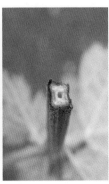

Round Angular Flanged Quadrangular

Root systems

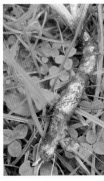 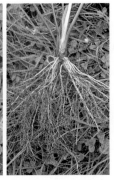

Taproot (single, thick, fleshy root) Fibrous roots (many, thin branching root)

Leaf veins

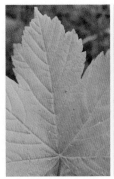 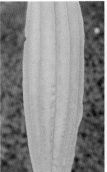 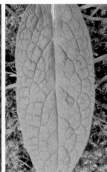

Palmate (hand-shaped veins) Parallel (longitudinal parallel veins) Pinnate (divided veins)

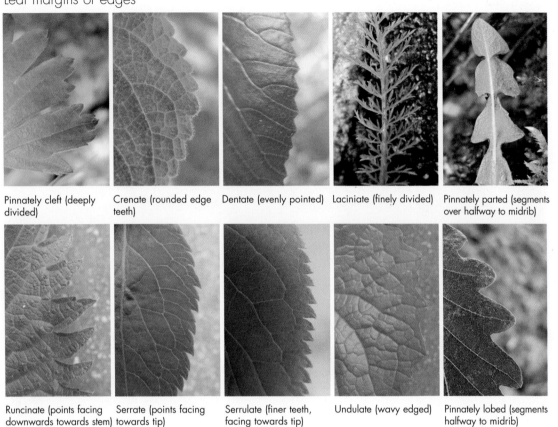

Pinnately cleft (deeply
divided)

Crenate (rounded edge
teeth)

Dentate (evenly pointed)

Laciniate (finely divided)

Pinnately parted (segments
over halfway to midrib)

Runcinate (points facing
downwards towards stem)

Serrate (points facing
towards tip)

Serrulate (finer teeth,
facing towards tip)

Undulate (wavy edged)

Pinnately lobed (segments
halfway to midrib)

How to identify plants

Leaf arrangements

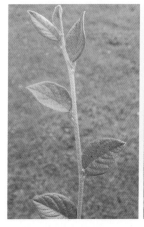

Alternate (arranged singly along stem)

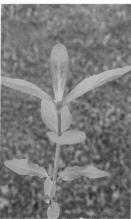

Decussate (rotating 90 degrees at each pair along stem)

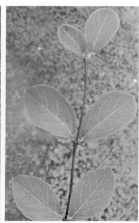

Opposite (in pairs along stem)

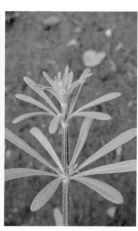

Whorled (three or more leaves around one point on stem)

Compound leaves

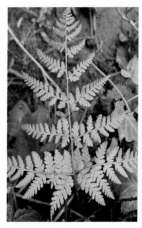

Bipinnate (leaflets on second rib division)

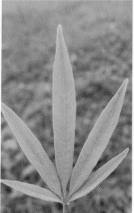

Palmate (leaflets arise from a central point)

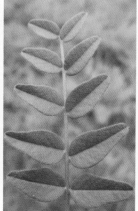

Pinnate even (even number of leaflets)

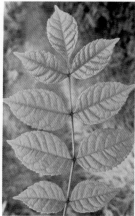

Pinnate uneven (uneven number of leaflets)

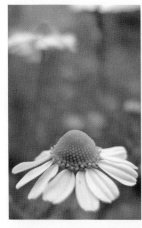

Capitulum (compact mass of stalkless flowers)

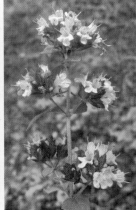

Panicle (branched stalks baring many flowers)

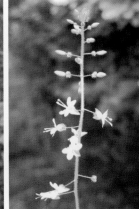

Raceme (short, single stalked flowers)

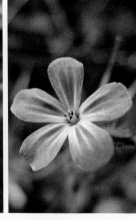

Solitary (stem baring single flower at its end)

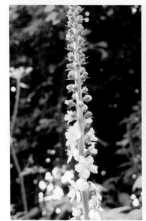

Spike (stem baring stalkless flowers)

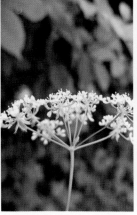

Umbel (many flower stalks all branching from same point)

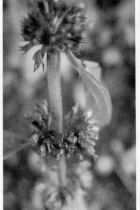

Whorl (flowers forming around stem)

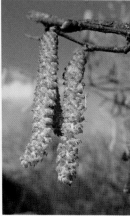

Catkin (cylindrical flower cluster, often drooping)

How to identify plants

Plant families

Plants are divided into different families depending on their basic structures. There are more than 200 plant families; those described here are ones mentioned in this book. Having an awareness of these basic family traits will aid identification when you are out foraging.

Aesculaceae
Trees with large palmate leaves and seeds with an eye-like spot.

Boraginaceae
The name comes from the Latin *burra*, meaning 'rough hair'; they are covered with stiff hairs on the stem and leaves, which are simple and alternate.

Caprifoliaceae
Bushes with pithy stems. The leaves are opposite and the flowers and berries are borne in pairs or bunches.

Caryophyllaceae
The flowers have petals that are split at the ends, and five sepals and petals.

Compositae
Plate-like flowers made up of a multitude of individual, tiny, tube-like flowers. Some of those flowers have over-large ray petals.

Cruciferae
Think of a crucifix or cross, as the flowers have four sepals, four petals and four long stamens with two short stamens deep in the flower. Seedpods grow in a spiral around the stem.

Equisetaceae
Spore-producing plants with rough, jointed stems.

Fagaceae
These are shrubs or trees that bear single nuts, often with scaly or prickly cases.

Fumariaceae
The flowers most commonly are irregular-shaped with two sepals and four petals.

Gramineae/Poaceae
Grassy plants with brittle nodules on the stems.

Hippocastanaceae
(See Aesculaceae)

Hypericaceae/Guttiferae
Plants with simple, opposite leaves and flowers with four or five sepals and petals.

Labiatae
The stems of these plants are square with leaves positioned opposite each other. These plants are often scented. Five fused sepals and petals make up the trumpet-like flowers. They have four stamens, two long and two short.

Liliaceae

Plants belonging to the onion sub family arise from mostly edible bulbs and characteristically feature small umbrella-like flowers.

Malvaceae

The flowers have five separate petals with stamens that have fused into a column around the pistil in the centre.

Papaveraceae

The flowers most commonly have petals in sets of four and many stamens.

Papilionaceae

The leaves are pinnate and the flowers have a distinctive shape that forms a banner with wings and a keel.

Plantaginaceae

Plants with parallel-veined leaves and long flower stalks bearing small, green flowers.

Polygonaceae

The flowers have no petals, but tiny, coloured sepals. The seeds are usually triangular.

Ranunculaceae

There are no strong patterns to identify the buttercup family except for a three-lobed pistil with hooked ends.

Rosaceae

These plants bear flowers with five sepals and five petals with many stamens. The leaves are usually serrated.

Rubiaceae

The leaves of these plants are whorled and the seeds are divided into two.

Salicaceae

Trees that grow in moist ground and have alternate leaves and catkin flowers.

Scrophulariaceae

The irregular-shaped flowers have three lower lobes and two upper ones, and many seeds in capsules.

Tiliaceae

Trees that have leaf-like bracts with clusters of flowers or seeds.

Urticaceae

These plants are usually hairy, like the nettle. They have flowers that hang in long strings from the leaf axils, with no petals.

Valerianaceae

Plants with basal, opposite leaves and tiny flowers. The roots are strongly scented.

Verbenaceae

The leaves are opposite and there are five of each of the flower parts: petals, stamens and sepals.

Violaceae

Plants with irregular-shaped flowers, such as those of pansies. They have exploding seedpods that scatter many seeds.

Viscaceae

Green plants that are parasitic on tree branches.

Plant families

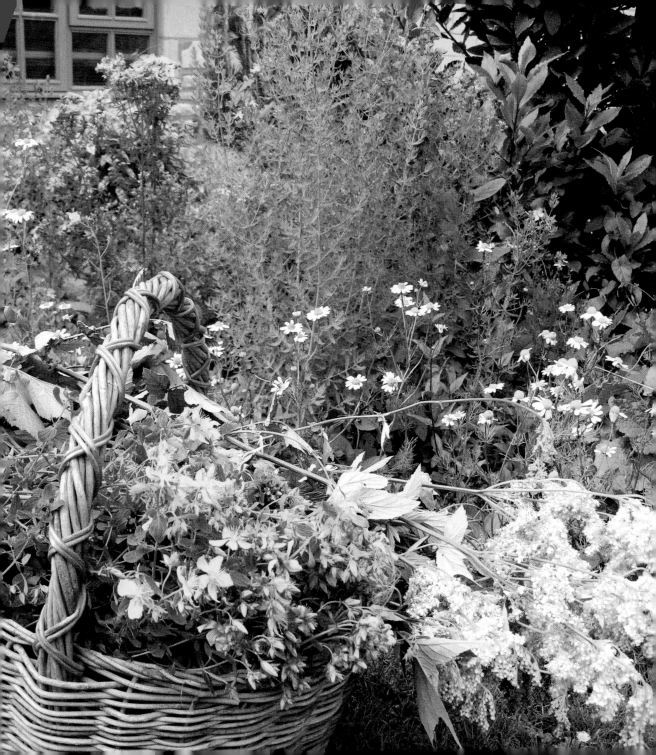

USING MEDICINAL PLANTS

Each person that uses medicinal plants will find his or her own favourite herbs and ways of preparing and taking them. When you become familiar with a plant – how it looks, tastes and with the effects it has on your body – you will find a way to use it that suits you best. Refine your skills, use your common sense and experiment. It is most important to realize that herbs treat people not ailments.

How herbs work

Herbal medicine uses natural plant constituents to help the human body in the process of healing. Their effects are not immediate, but they work with the body's own systems to promote long-lasting health.

All plants contain chemical compounds that they produce as part of their metabolism. These include: primary metabolites that are involved in providing energy for growth and reproduction, such as sugars and fats; and secondary metabolites that are produced to help the plant defend itself against attack from predators and disease. All of these metabolites, called constituents, provide useful substances that can be

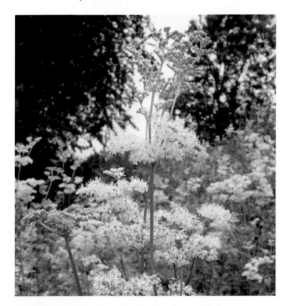

Meadowsweet contains salicylate that has anti-inflammatory effects on the body.

utilized by the body to produce a healing response to imbalances that manifest as symptoms of disease.

Science is beginning to investigate these healing constituents and observe how they affect the body at a cellular level, but it is often still at a loss to explain how many plants work, despite a demonstrable action. They also often seem to have an action greater than that expected from the individual actions of the constituents. This is known as synergy, the importance of which is only just beginning to be understood. There is also a synergy that occurs when combining herbs for medicine, allowing treatment to be tailored to individuals. This makes the effectiveness of herbal medicines difficult to measure in current testing, which is why there is much conflicting evidence on the efficacy of herbs. It is here that traditional and ethnobotanical knowledge is invaluable. These remedies simply would not have continued to be used if they were not effective. Furthermore, they would not be found being used in similar ways by indigenous people spread widely around the world.

How herbs affect the body

Herbs basically work in three main ways: stimulation, nutrition and elimination. These actions do not suppress symptoms – they are supporting what the body is trying to do naturally. Herbal medicines take time to work as they facilitate the body to heal itself. Chronic ailments may take a long time to respond as they have taken a long time to develop, a rough guide being one month per year of the condition. Acute ailments often respond quite quickly and the benefit is usually felt in a few days. However, it is important to consider what made the body susceptible to the illness.

Stimulation

Some constituents have direct effects on the actions of the body by stimulating them to act in a certain way, in the same way as orthodox drugs. However, these powerful substances usually occur in much smaller concentrations in herbs and they are buffered by the other constituents in that plant. For example, meadowsweet (see page 169) contains salicylate, the chemical from which aspirin was developed, which in a concentrated form is an irritant to the lining of the digestive tract. Meadowsweet is good for digestive irritation, however, because it also contains substances that soothe and tone the membranes, while the salicylate has an anti-inflammatory effect.

Nutrition

Herbs are like foods – they provide essential nutrition to enable the body to function efficiently. Different herbs have an affinity with different areas of the body. This is because they contain substances that are required for normal function in that area.

Elimination

Many herbs have cleansing effects that increase elimination of by-products of metabolism from the body. The routes of elimination are urination (diuretics), bowels (laxatives), sweating (diaphoretics) and breathing (expectorants).

Actions of herbs

Herbs can be grouped by their actions. When combining herbs for treatment identify the herbal actions that the body requires to aid it in healing. For example, urine infection requires an antiseptic herb (wild thyme) to fight the infection, a demulcent herb (mallow) to soothe the inflammation and relieve pain and a diuretic herb (couch grass) to flush out the accumulated waste. There are many herbs within each group described overleaf, and they often cross over in their actions.

A holistic approach

When treating illness with herbal medicine, it is imperative to consider all aspects of the person's life. The body is constantly striving to achieve a balance between burning energy and creating energy in response to its environment. Diet, nutrition, emotional and spiritual well-being, environment and lifestyle are the foundations of health. Illness arises as a result of an imbalance in one or more of these factors and the body's attempts to adjust to it.

Rather than treating just the specific symptoms of an illness, always focus on treating the whole person. When deciding which herbs to take, consider all of the above factors and try to understand what the body requires to enhance its natural functions. Then it becomes clear which herbs are appropriate to address the root of the problem rather than the symptoms.

Using medicinal plants

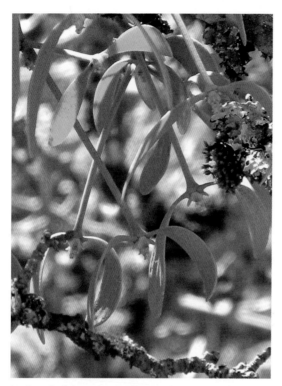

Mistletoe herb has relaxant effects on the nervous system affecting the blood vessels.

Astringents

Astringents tone up relaxed tissue, reduce secretion of mucous membranes and can help reduce bleeding. Tannins are the active constituents here – these create the taste that dries your mouth, such as strong black tea. Astringent herbs include horse chestnut (see page 38), wood avens (see page 44), oak (see page 47), pilewort (see page 50), horsetail (see page 67), yarrow (see page 84), agrimony (see page 87), shepherd's purse (see page 131) golden rod (see page 146), ground ivy (see page 175) and white deadnettle (see page 181).

Relaxants

Relaxants reduce tension in tissues by working on the nervous system, relaxing hollow organs and blood vessels. Secretions increase from mucous membranes and from sweat glands. Relaxant herbs are lime (see page 56), mistletoe (see page 59), valerian (see page 79), yarrow (see page 84), oat (see page 93), chamomile (see page 102), mugwort (see page 128), St John's wort (see page 137), vervain (see page 161), hop (see page 178), mint (see page 198) and wood betony (see page 111).

Bitters

These work through their taste, stimulating the release of the hormone gastrin. Gastrin increases the release of all digestive enzymes from the stomach, liver and pancreas. Bitters are used for poor appetite and sluggish bowels, infection (as they increase white cells) and diabetes. They are useful for digestive fullness and flatulence as they reduce fermentation in the gut. Bitter herbs include agrimony (see page 87), fumitory (see page 99), yellow dock (see page 108), dandelion root (see page 114), burdock (see page 125) and hop (see page 178).

Stimulants

These increase circulation, energy and vitality. They are usually very warming. They stimulate the nervous system and therefore reflexes. Stimulant herbs include yarrow (see page 84) and horseradish (see page 122).

Demulcents

These plants contain thick, viscous sap. They are used for soothing inflamed mucous membranes, coating them in a thick healing 'plaster' and stimulating increased production of mucus. Examples of plants in this group are mallow (see page 64), comfrey (see page 76), plantain (see page 105) and mullein (see page 158).

Expectorants
These plants are known as local stimulants that work on the respiratory tract by liquefying sticky, thick mucus and aiding its expulsion from the lungs. They also constrict the blood vessels of the nose, reducing congestion. Plants belonging to this group include wild garlic (see page 41), elecampane (see page 140), coltsfoot (see page 152), mint (see page 198), wild thyme (see page 204) and sweet violet (see page 207).

Nervines
These herbs all have an affinity for the nervous system. They are either stimulating or relaxing and are often nourishing and restorative. They include lime (see page 56), oat (see page 93), St John's wort (see page 137), vervain (see page 161) and wood betony (see page 111).

Diuretics
The plants included in this group increase the flow of urine and promote cleansing via the kidneys and bladder. They include couch grass (see page 90), dandelion leaf (see page 114), golden rod (see page 146) and nettle (see page 155).

Diaphoretics
These herbs induce sweating and are used in fevers and in the treatment of disordered circulation; they may also be relaxing or stimulating. They include lime (see page 56), yarrow (see page 84), horseradish (see page 122) and elderflower (see page 184).

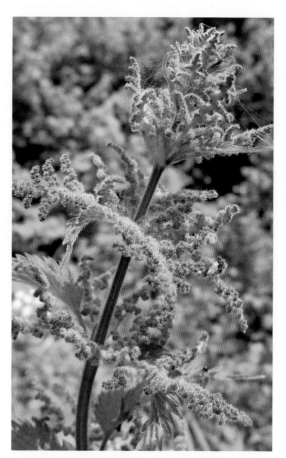

Nettles are considered diuretic but they also have other invaluable actions on the body.

Laxatives
There are bulking laxatives such as plantain seeds (see page 105) and stimulant laxatives that irritate the bowel to produce the urge to defecate, such as yellow dock (see page 108). Stimulant laxatives are often given with a carminative (a substance that relieves flatulence) to prevent pain in the bowels. Bitter liver herbs can also improve bowel function.

Preparing herbs

Correct preparation of herbs is an important step to ensure that the healing power of the herb is not lost or destroyed, but its therapeutic action is enhanced by the method of extraction by making it easily ingested or applied and absorbed.

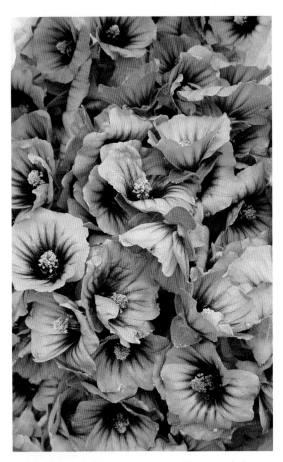

Mallow flowers make a stunning, tasty addition to salads, or their properties may be preserved into a soothing syrup.

Whole plants

If any stems or leaves have mud on them, wipe it off with a damp cloth. Do not wash them. Spread out the plants and leave for an hour or so to let any creatures escape. Chop into 2 cm (3/4 in) pieces for tincturing. For drying, bunch together six stems, tie them up by the stems with rubber bands and hang them upside down, preferably in a dark and airy place. When dry, the stems should be brittle and snap cleanly but the colour of the leaves and flowers should be largely preserved. Strip off the leaves and flowers and cut up the stems into 5 mm (1/5 in) lengths.

Roots

Put roots in water for an hour to soak and use a brush to clean off any mud. Keep rinsing smaller roots until the water runs clean. For large quantities of roots, put them in a clean cotton pillowcase, tie it shut with string and run it through a rinse cycle in the washing machine (run a rinse cycle on empty first to remove any washing residues). Cut into 1–2 cm (1/2–3/4 in) pieces before tincturing or drying.

To dry, spread the pieces of root on trays or clean sheets of paper and leave in a warm, dry, well-ventilated place until they become dry to the touch and brittle (ideally 7–10 days). Alternatively, place them in a warm oven on its lowest setting for a few hours.

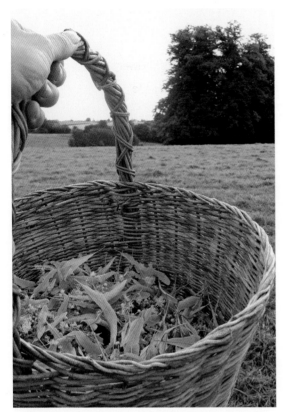

Limeflowers develop a stronger scent as they dry and make a fragrant, calming infusion.

Leaves

Wipe off any mud with a damp cloth. Chop up leaves for tinctures. To dry, spread them on trays or clean sheets of paper in a single layer and put them in a warm, dry, well-ventilated place, out of direct sunlight, for a few days. Ideally, they should be brittle but the colour should be mainly preserved.

Flowers

Flowers rarely need cleaning. Chop large flowers for tinctures and dry as for leaves (see above).

Seeds

Seeds should already be dry when harvested.

Berries

Berries rarely need cleaning and can be tinctured whole, or slightly crushed. To dry, spread berries out on trays and leave in a warm dry, well-ventilated place until totally dry (ideally 7–10 days), or place in an oven on its lowest setting for a few hours.

Sap

Apply sap directly from the plant to the affected area.

Preparing herbs

Bark

Brush bark to remove loose debris and moss or lichens. Cut into approximately 1–2 cm ($^1/_2$–$^3/_4$ in) pieces before tincturing or drying.

To dry bark, spread the pieces on trays or clean sheets of paper and leave in a warm, dry, well-ventilated place until they become dry to the touch and brittle (ideally 7–10 days). Alternatively, place them in a warm oven on its lowest setting for a few hours.

Storing herbs

Store dried herbs in a cool, dry, dark place in airtight jars. Label each jar with details such as what the herb is, when and where it was picked, and when it was put in the jar. Dried stems, leaves and flowers will keep for up to a year. Roots, berries and bark will keep for 2–3 years.

How to take herbs

The simplest way of making the healing properties of a herb available to the body is to use it raw either by eating it or applying it directly to the skin. Other methods of taking herbs involve making infusions, decoctions, tinctures, infused oils, salves, ointments and syrups.

Herbs as food

In spring, many herbs can be eaten raw; try nibbling delicate, tender buds, leaves and flowers of medicinal plants while on a walk, or gather them and add them to salads (but see page 15 regarding poisonous plants). Hawthorn leaves and flowers, wild garlic leaves and flowers, chickweed, dandelion, ground ivy, hop shoots, meadowsweet, mint, plantain, red clover flowers, sweet violet leaves and flowers, white deadnettle flowers and thyme are all tasty when raw.

Some herbs need to be cooked to be palatable. They may be steamed or stir-fried as a vegetable or added into soups, stews or omelettes. Nettles, wild garlic, burdock root, dandelion leaves and root, elderflowers and berries, hop shoots, mallow root and milk thistle shoots are all delicious when cooked and eaten.

The fresh sap of some plants, such as dandelion and celandine, is used topically for the treatment of skin conditions. Simple poultices are useful while in the field. Pick some clean, dry leaves and rub them hard to soften and draw moisture out. Then place over the affected area and hold or bind in place and change every hour. A very basic poultice is a 'spit poultice', made by chewing up a few leaves of the herb and applying to the area. Ensure you know the plant is safe first. Chickweed, plantain, comfrey, dock, yarrow and daisy are useful topically in their raw state.

Infusions

Infusions are used for leaves and flowers. Use them topically as a wash or in a bath, as a douche or enema, or they can be drunk hot or cold or used as a gargle or mouthwash. The infused herbs can also be put between gauze and used as a poultice. Herbs used for drinking are dependent on personal taste – some herbs make very pleasant-tasting teas that can be included in daily life as a general health tonic or for long-term treatment in chronic ailments. Many herbs have a bitter flavour that some people might find unpalatable but others enjoy. It is common to enjoy the taste of a herb that your body needs. It is also

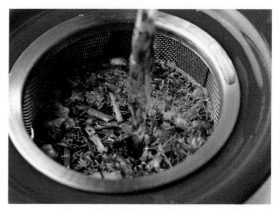

Pleasant-tasting infusions of herbs can be incorporated into your daily routine as therapeutic substitutes for tea and coffee.

common suddenly to find the same herb distasteful when the body no longer requires it.

Experiment with combinations of herbs. Consider the different actions needed from each herb: anti-infectious, soothing, relaxing and toning. Herbs containing mucilage, such as mallow and comfrey, need to be cold infused as hot water destroys mucilage. Drink hot infusions to help induce sweating and cooling in fevers. Try drinking cooled infusions to stimulate urination.

Method Add 25 g (1 oz) dried herb or 50 g (2 oz) fresh herb to 600 ml (1 pint) boiling water. A china tea ball holds a dose adequate for a mug of herbal tea. Cover and leave to infuse for ten minutes. Strain and drink.

Dose 200 ml (7 fl oz) three times a day for chronic ailments; 200 ml (7 fl oz) every two hours for acute conditions.

Use by Infusions will keep well in the refrigerator for 24 hours.

Decoctions

A decoction is used for roots, berries and bark, and can be used in the same ways as infusions.

Method Use the same proportions as for an infusion. Place the herb in a pan with a lid and bring to the boil and simmer for 20 minutes.

Dose 200 ml (7 fl oz) three times a day for chronic ailments; 200 ml (7 fl oz) every two hours for acute conditions.

Use by Decoctions keep in the refrigerator for 24 hours.

Tinctures

Alcohol is a good preservative for herbs. Alcohol will dissolve and extract the active substances and preserve them. Fresh herb tinctures yield more on pressing than dried herb tinctures.

A minimum of 25 per cent alcohol is required to preserve and inhibit the growth of unwanted organisms. Herbalists use ethanol, which is 96 per cent, and dilute it with water to the concentration they require, depending on the active constituents they wish to extract. For making home tinctures, vodka, at 37–40 per cent alcohol, is adequate for most herbs. Resinous herbs (myrrh, frankincense, hops) need 90 per cent alcohol to dissolve them. For plants with a high water content, allowing them to wilt overnight will encourage water to evaporate off and ensure a stronger final alcohol content and less chance of fermentation.

Method **Fresh herb:** use 1 part herb to 2 parts vodka – for example, 100 g (4 oz) herb to 200 ml (7 fl oz) vodka. **Dried herb:** use 1 part herb to 5 parts vodka – for example, 100 g (4 oz) dried herb to 500 ml (17 fl oz) vodka.

Put the herbs into a large, clean jar and pour over the vodka; seal and store in a cool, dark place for two weeks, shaking occasionally. Strain through a muslin cloth and press out all the liquid. Bottle and label with name and date.

Dose 1 teaspoon three times a day, taken in a little water or juice, for chronic ailments. 1 teaspoon every two hours, in water, for acute ailments, for eight doses then three times a day until better.

Use by Tinctures can be kept for up to three years, and even longer if they are stored in a cool, dark place and the bottle is not opened regularly. They can be decanted into smaller bottles as required.

Infused oils

Infusing herbs in sunflower or grapeseed oil will extract and preserve the properties of some plants so they may be used directly on the skin. Use this method

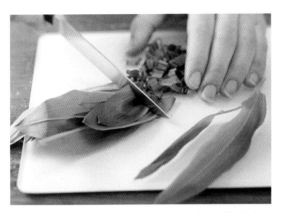

Maintain high standards of hygiene in the making of herbal remedies by keeping certain utensils only for herb preparation.

for herbs with aromatic or skin-healing qualities, such as chamomile, chickweed, comfrey, St John's wort flowers, mullein flowers, yarrow and plantain, or elderflowers.

Sun method Use this for St John's wort and mullein flowers, as heat would destroy the active constituents. Pick the flowers on a dry day before the sun gets too hot. Place in a clean, dry jar and pour on sunflower or grapeseed oil to cover the flowers. Put the lid on and leave on a sunny windowledge, shaking every day or so. Leave for two weeks. Strain off the oil and label.

Heat method Use this for other herbs. Gather the plant on a dry day and leave to wilt for a few hours so that some of the water evaporates out. Make a bain-marie with a bowl over a saucepan of water so the base of the bowl is immersed in the water. Chop up any large leaves. Put half the herbs into the bowl and pour over sunflower or grapeseed oil to cover them. Turn on the heat and bring the water up to a simmer. Leave the herbs to infuse in the oil for two hours. Strain the oil out, pour it back onto a fresh batch of wilted herb and repeat the infusion. Strain and leave to settle for a few hours. Pour off and discard any water and plant residue that has separated out or it will go mouldy and make the oil rancid. Bottle and label.

Dose Apply the oil to the affected area up to four times a day.

Use by Infused oils will usually keep for one year. Dispose of the oil if it smells rancid or develops mould.

Ointments and salves

Ointments and salves combine infused oils with beeswax to provide a waterproof moisturizing barrier for the skin that delivers the herb's healing qualities.

Method To make 25 g (1 oz) soft set salve, measure out 25 ml (1 fl oz) of the chosen infused oil. Put the oil in a pan over a gentle heat and add 5 g (1/4 oz) beeswax. When it has melted, dip in a cold teaspoon to check setting consistency. Add more beeswax if a harder salve is required. Pour into the jar and label.

Dose Cover the affected area up to three times a day.

Use by Salves keep for about a year; if it smells good it remains useful and if it smells rancid dispose of it.

Syrups

These are useful for coughs and sore throats, and for treating children because they taste nice. They also soothe irritated membranes they come into contact with and deliver the herb's healing properties directly to the place that needs them.

Method Infuse or decoct your herbs. Strain and reduce by slowly simmering the resulting liquid to a third of its volume. For every 200 ml (7 fl oz) of liquid, add 400 ml (14 fl oz) honey or 150 g (5 oz) sugar of your choice. Stir until dissolved, bottle and label. Store in the refrigerator.

Dose Take 1–2 teaspoons every two hours for acute coughs, or four times a day for chronic coughs.

Use by Six months. Discard if mould appears.

Self-treatment essentials

Do not take herbs for long periods at therapeutic doses if you do not need them. If you are unwell and try a remedy and do not have any improvement after a few weeks then seek expert advice from a medical herbalist. If you are uncertain in any way about treating yourself then seek out a medical herbalist (www.nimh.org.uk). Most herbalists run walks and talks and short courses so you can build up your knowledge under the direct instruction of an experienced expert.

Doses and measurements

When smaller than standard doses are used for specific herbs it is important to measure them accurately. A syringe or small measuring cylinder can be obtained from most pharmacies. When parts are described, it is easiest to make the combination up to 175 g (6 oz) for dried herbs (enough for a week, at 25 g (1 oz) infused per day) or 100 ml (3^1/$_2$ fl oz) for tinctures (enough for a week at 1 teaspoon (5 ml) three times a day).

Treating babies and children

Children's illnesses are usually mild and will quickly resolve themselves, even though the symptoms may sometimes appear alarming, with high temperatures and fever. They have a faster metabolism than adults and illness can develop rapidly. Herbs may be used as gentle remedies for children, although they may require plenty of sweetening. (Do not give honey to children under 1 year, or honey that is unpasteurized to children under 2 years.) Have children under the age of 4 years treated by a qualified medical herbalist.

Warning You must seek professional help in the following cases:

* There is severe diarrhoea or vomiting, or mild diarrhoea that lasts for more than 12 hours.
* Temperature is above 39°C (102°F) for more than two hours.
* There are convulsions, breathing problems or unusual drowsiness.
* There is an unusual, high-pitched cry.

Doses

* Breastfed babies under three months of age: herbs will reach them via the breast milk.
* Chamomile is a gentle and safe remedy for all children that can be successfully used to settle most common children's ailments.

Infusion doses:

* 4–5 years: 50 ml (2 fl oz) three times a day
* 6–8 years: 100 ml (3^1/$_2$ fl oz) three times a day
* 8–10 years: 150 ml (^{1}/$_4$ pint) three times a day
* 10 years and over: 200 ml (7 fl oz) three times a day

Tincture doses:

* 4–5 years: 1.5 ml three times a day.
* 6–8 years: 2.5 ml three times a day.
* 8–10 years: 3.5 ml three times a day.
* 10 years and over: 5 ml three times a day.

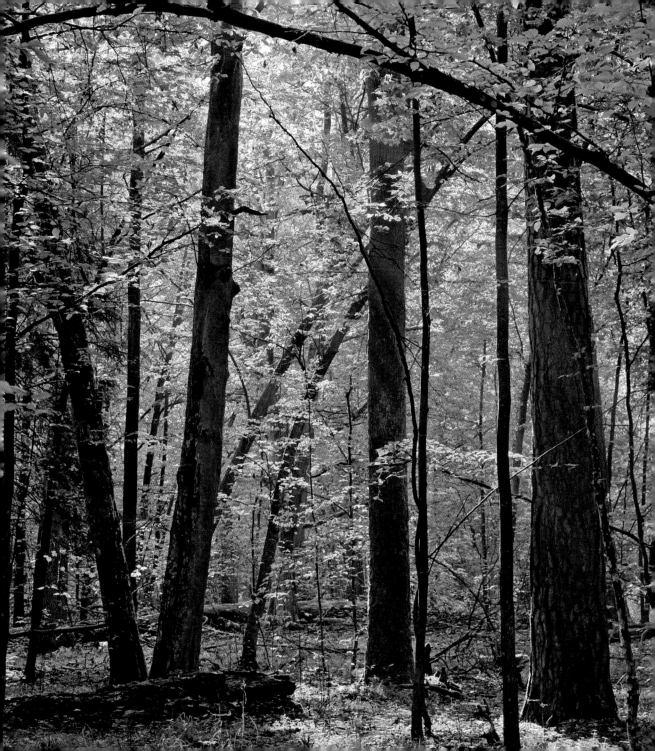

WOODLAND PLANTS

A walk in the woods is always a magical experience, but woodlands also harbour an abundance of medicinal plants, both in the trees themselves and in the smaller plants that like to grow in their shadow. When you spend time harvesting here, you are in a place of tranquil healing that lightens the spirit with the sound of bird song and shelters you from the elements of rain, wind and sun.

Aesculus hippocastanum

Horse chestnut

conkers

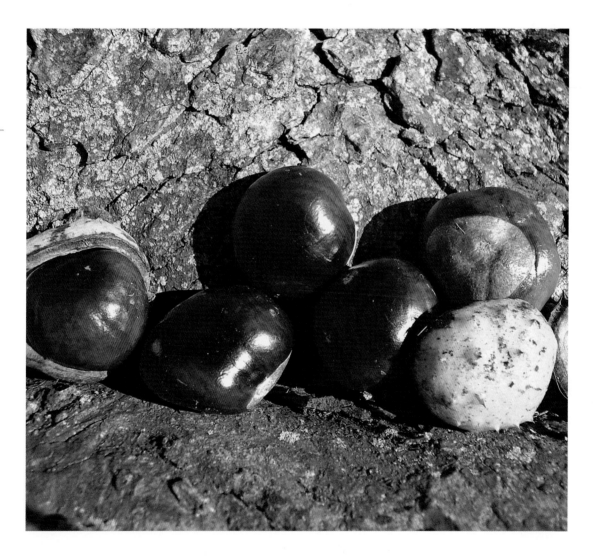

Fact and folklore

The horse chestnut is an elegant, ornamental tree often grown in parks and gardens. It is well known for its shiny, brown seeds or 'conkers' (found within prickly seed cases), which children like to play with. When the seed is ground and mixed with water, the saponins it contains make a soapy foam and the water was traditionally used to wash clothes. The seed is also rich in tannins, and the combination of these constituents is tonic for the veins. It will tighten up weak venous walls and valves, reducing the size of varicose veins in the legs and also in haemorrhoids (piles). The bark has similar but milder properties.

What to look for

This large tree, which grows to 30 m (100 ft), bears large, brown, sticky leaf-buds in the early spring, from which the leaves unfurl. The leaves are light green and have 5–7 oval leaflets that resemble the shape of a hand. The white and pink flowers are borne on large pyramid-shaped bunches, 15–30 cm (6–12 in) long. The round, brown seeds are encased in prickly green shells that turn brown when ripe. These shells split into 3–4 sections when they drop from the tree and bear 1–2 seeds.

Can be mistaken for

Sweet chestnut (*Castanea sativa*) has similar seed casings, but they are densely prickled and the seeds are pointed at one end. The leaves are pointed and oval, with serrated edges.

Where to look

Horse chestnut is widely cultivated in parks and gardens around Europe and also found growing wild in meadows and woodland.

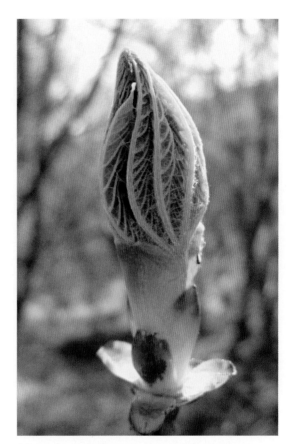

A horse chestnut leaf emerging from its sticky covering. The leaves have similar but milder actions than the conkers.

When to look for it

The leaves open in April, flowers appear in May and it drops the 'conkers' in September.

What to harvest

The bark, leaves and conkers.

What is it good for?

Haemorrhoids (piles) • Varicose veins

Horse chestnut

How to use it

The fresh seeds are quite toxic and irritant to the digestive tract. Collect, then peel the seeds and chop them into large lumps; dry these and roughly grind them before tincturing. Take small doses of 1–2 ml (see page 35) of the tincture with food to protect the digestive tract from the potentially irritating effects. Use a decoction of the dried seeds as a lotion or compress for varicose veins or haemorrhoids (piles). The decoction is so unpalatable as to make it difficult to drink in any therapeutic quantity.

Cautions

Saponins break up red blood cells when they come into contact with them, so may cause haemolytic anaemia. However, they are poorly absorbed in the digestive tract and do not really come into contact with the blood stream. Therefore, do not take if you have a history of gastritis, heartburn or gastrointestinal ulceration or bleeding, or apply to areas of broken skin where they may be absorbed into the blood stream. Do not take during pregnancy. Do not use in combination with anticoagulant medication. Do not use fresh seeds. They are not edible like sweet chestnut (*Castanea sativa*). Do not use tannin rich herbs for longer than two weeks at a time. It is advised to take this herb with the supervision of a medical herbalist.

Combines well with

Dandelion leaf tincture (see page 114) for leg oedema or ankle swelling due to varicose veins
Yarrow (see page 84) and oak (see page 47) as an infusion for use as a compress for haemorrhoids (piles)

Forager's checklist

* **Large deciduous tree**
* **Widely cultivated**
* **Prickly-cased seeds or conkers**
* **Seeds are used**
* **Tonic for the veins**
* **30 m (100 ft) high**
* **Family: Hippocastanaceae/Aesculaceae**

Try it in conker vein lotion

Measure 75 ml (3 fl oz) yarrow infused oil. Add 25 ml (1 fl oz) of horsechestnut tincture followed by 20 drops of cypress essential oil (optional). Shake the mixture well before use. Apply the lotion directly to varicose veins two times a day. This lotion will keep for up to a year.

Woodland plants

Allium ursinum
Wild garlic
ramsons, bear's garlic

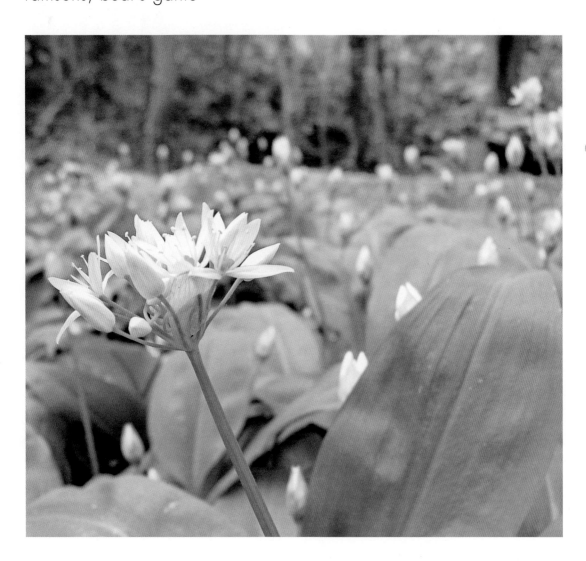

Fact and folklore

Carpeting woodland and shaded groves in early spring, wild garlic has been a traditional pot herb for hundreds of years. It is said that when the devil followed man from the Garden of Eden garlic grew where he put his right foot and onion where he put his left one. It is called 'bear's garlic' and *ursinum* because bears love to eat it.

Cooking reduces its potency; raw cultivated garlic has been shown to reduce total cholesterol levels by up to 19 per cent. It also thins the blood and is useful when the blood clots too easily. It is restorative on the blood vessel walls and therefore useful for high blood pressure and atherosclerosis. Garlic is a potent anti-septic and an effective treatment for colds, sore throats, sinusitis, catarrh and chest infections. The anti-infective property comes from the volatile oil that is excreted via the lungs, which is why it is smelt on the breath. It is a stimulating expectorant and thins thick mucus. It also stimulates the immune system, enabling the body to fight infections.

What to look for

Wild garlic grows from an underground bulb, to 25 cm (10 in) high. Large, pointed, oval leaves, 10–20 cm (4–8 in) long, appear in clumps and smell strongly of garlic. The flowers grow at the top of a long stem, bearing a mass of white, star-like flowers, each with five petals.

Can be mistaken for

Growing at the same time and in the same places are the leaves of cuckoo pint (*Arum maculatum*); these are similar in colour but have distinct, arrow-shaped leaves that do not smell of garlic. Cultivated garlic has the same but stronger properties.

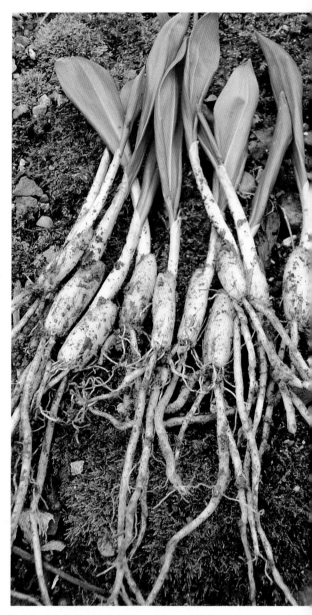

Wild garlic bulbs may be used in the same way as cultivated garlic; it has milder medicinal properties and flavour.

Where to look

Wild garlic likes damp soil and grows in shaded copses, banks, hedgerows and woodland.

When to look for it

The leaves and flowers appear from March to May. Harvest the bulbs in autumn or early spring.

What to harvest

The leaves, flowers and bulb.

What is it good for?

Boils • Cold sores • Conjunctivitis • Cramp • Bronchitis • Catarrh • Colds • Coughs • Earache • Flu • Sinusitis • Sore throat • Atherosclerosis • Chilblains • High cholesterol • High blood pressure • Fungal infections • Infection • Diverticular disease • Worms

How to use it

The leaves are best eaten fresh in the spring, either lightly cooked in an omelette or as a leaf herb in salads or sandwiches. The flowers make a pretty garnish. The bulb may be dug up in early spring, before the leaves are fully grown, or in the autumn and used in cooking as for cultivated garlic bulbs. Eat the leaves freely throughout the day and eat the bulbs chopped on a slice of toast at least three times a day, for acute conditions. The leaves also make delicious wild garlic pesto when blended with pine nuts, olive oil and Parmesan cheese. Make a fresh tincture of the whole plant to preserve all its properties.

Cautions

Do not use in combination with any orthodox anticoagulants. Do not take if you suffer from a bleeding condition.

Combines well with

Wild thyme (see page 204) for infections
Lime (see page 56) for high cholesterol

Try it in garlic cough-and-catarrh honey

Take six wild garlic bulbs and chop each into three pieces. Put them in a jar and cover them with honey. Leave for a few hours or overnight before using the honey. The garlic can be left in. If using cultivated garlic, use fewer bulbs as they are stronger. Doses are:

- 4–6 years: $1/2$ teaspoon every 4 hours
- 7–10 years: 1 teaspoon every 4 hours
- Over 10 years: 1 teaspoon every 2 hours

Do not give to children under 2 years (see page 35). Keep in the refrigerator for six months.

Wild garlic

Forager's checklist

❋ **Bulbous plant**

❋ **Common woodland plant**

❋ **Leaves make delicious spring greens**

❋ **Harvest the bulb in autumn or early spring**

❋ **Dense growth of green leaves and white, star-like flowers**

❋ **Distinct garlic smell**

❋ **Powerful antibiotic**

❋ **25 cm (10 in) high**

❋ **Family: Liliaceae**

Geum urbanum

Wood avens

herba benedicta, herb bennet, clove root

Woodland plants

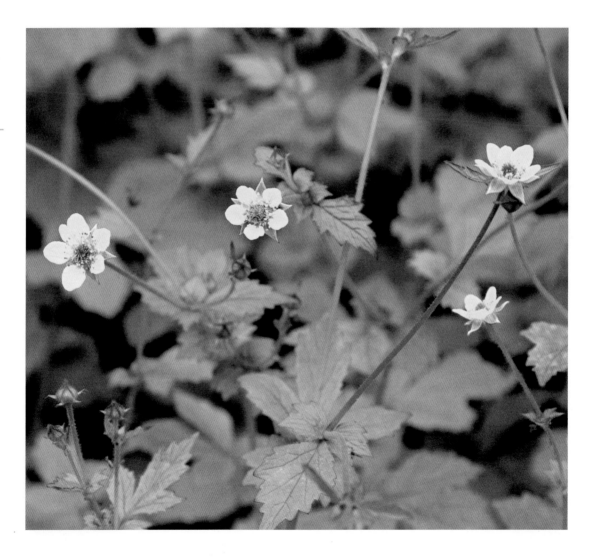

Fact and folklore

Wood avens was considered a very holy plant because the leaves are trifoliate (having three parts) and are therefore thought to represent the Trinity, and the five petals of the flowers were taken to represent the five wounds of Christ. The alternative name 'herb bennet' is a corruption of 'herba benedicta' ('blessed herb'). The plant was thought to protect against evil when worn as an amulet.

It was traditionally used to flavour ale – a small bag of the fresh root was included into fermenting casks to impart a delicate taste of cloves. Before the spice trade began importing cloves into Europe and Britain, wood avens would have been a prime remedy as an antiseptic herb for mucous membranes of the digestive tract. It is rich in tannins that tighten up congested membranes that are over-secreting mucus.

What to look for

Long slender stems, 30–40 cm (12–16 in) high, end in a three-part leaf with finely serrated edges. The yellow, five-petalled flowers, only 3–5 mm ($1/8$–$1/4$ in) across, appear at the top of the stems. The seedhead is more noticeable and grows into a round, hooked bur, 5 mm ($1/4$ in) in diameter, which is green with red hues.

Can be mistaken for

Water avens (*Geum rivale*) has red flowers. A cross between wood avens and water avens has also been identified, with similar medicinal properties. The main distinguishing feature of wood avens is the mild, clove-scented root.

Where to look

Wood avens grows throughout Europe in woodland, shady hedgerows and on damp, grassy banks.

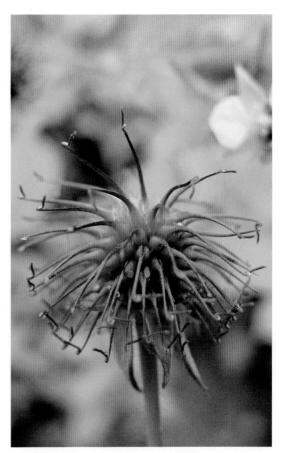

The seedheads of wood avens are a particularly distinctive, identifying feature of the plant.

When to look for it

You may find wood avens growing all year round in milder climates. It flowers from May to September.

What to harvest

The root in the early spring, at the beginning of the growing season, or in the autumn when the plant has died back.

Wood avens

What is it good for?
Gums and teeth • Mouth ulcers • Sore throat • Fungal infections • Diarrhoea • Irritable bowel syndrome (IBS)

How to use it
Use the tincture in a small amount of water as a mouthwash. Dilute it in larger quantities of warm water and take regularly for treating diarrhoea, either from an infective origin or from irritable or inflammatory bowel disease. The root when chewed is quite pleasant-tasting, with the astringent flavour of cloves. It can be used in this way either fresh or dried. The dried root can be decocted but the properties are reduced by this method of extraction.

Cautions
None.

Combines well with
Shepherd's purse (see page 131) and plantain (see page 105) for inflammatory bowel disease
Mallow (see page 64) and wild thyme (see page 204) for a sore throat

Try it in avens mouthwash
Mix together 40 ml (1^1/$_2$ fl oz) wood avens tincture, 30 ml (1^1/$_4$ fl oz) wild thyme tincture and 20 ml (^{3}/$_4$ fl oz) silverweed or oak bark tincture and 10 ml (2 teaspoons) of vegetable glycerine, which you can buy in a pharmacy, in a 100 ml (3^1/$_2$ fl oz) bottle. Use 10 ml (2 teaspoons) of this mix in a little water, twice a day after brushing teeth, as a mouthwash, for bleeding gums or gum disease. It will help to combat any infection and will also tone up spongy gums. It will keep in the refrigerator for up to three years.

Forager's checklist
* **Perennial herb**
* **Widely distributed**
* **Root smells faintly of cloves**
* **Antiseptic mucous membrane tonic**
* **Prefers shady places**
* **Fresh root is most potent**
* **Long growing season**
* **30–40 cm (12–16 in) high and 30 cm (12 in) wide**
* **Family: Rosaceae**

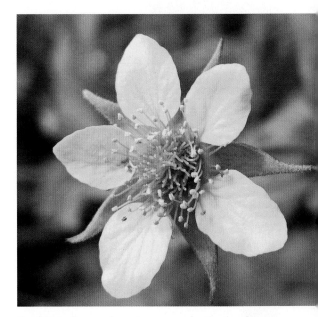

The delicate flowers of wood avens are short-lived and soon give way to the attractive red-hued seedheads.

Quercus robur

Oak

tanner's bark

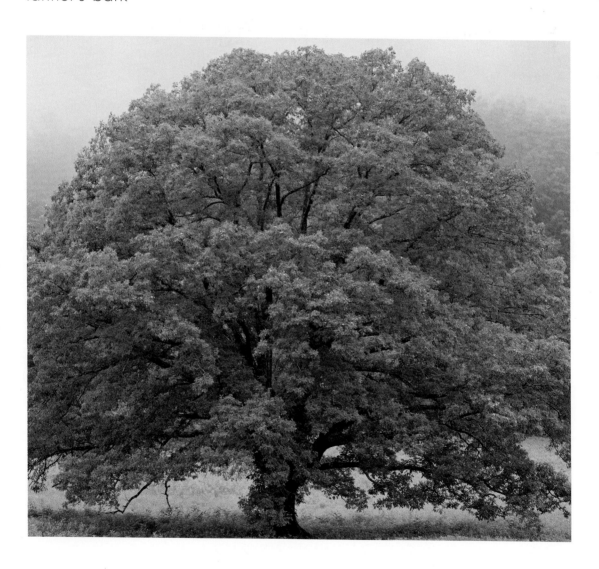

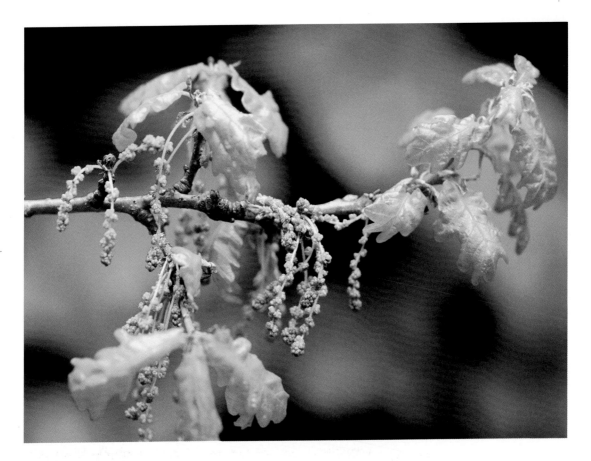

Fact and folklore

Oak trees live for centuries and there are records of specific trees living for well over a thousand years. The wood is extremely hard and durable, making it highly prized for building and cabinet-making; for centuries, ships were built from oak. The bark yields a dye of varying colours, depending on the fixative used, and it was also used for tanning leather. The bark is used medicinally for its astringent properties owing to the high tannin content. It is used to tone up relaxed membranes with excess discharge.

The catkin flowers of the oak emerge at the same time as the leaves in the early spring.

What to look for

The bark of an oak tree is brown-grey and deeply fissured in vertical, wavy, broken lines. The leaves are 8–10 cm (3^1/$_2$–4 in) long and have wavy edges. The seeds or acorns are recognizable as little rough-surfaced cups that each contain an oval, shiny, green-brown nut. Mature oak trees can grow up to 25 m (80 ft) high.

Can be mistaken for
There are several other species of oak (*Quercus* spp.), but the barks all have the same qualities.

Where to look
Oak grows in fields, woodland and parks.

When to look for it
It is a deciduous tree. In spring, look for boughs from young trees that have been snapped off in a storm.

What to harvest
The bark from younger trees.

What is it good for?
Gums and teeth • Catarrh • Sore throat • Bleeding • Haemorrhoids (piles) • Nosebleed • Varicose veins • Diarrhoea

How to use it
Dry the bark and use for weak decoctions ($1/2$ standard dose) for internal use, compresses and mouthwashes. Add the decoction to baths or washes for weeping skin conditions. Make the fresh bark into a tincture for small doses of 1–2 ml (see page 35) in combination with other herbs. Grind the bark into a fine powder and use a tiny pinch as a snuff twice a day for nasal polyps.

Cautions
Oak is a strong astringent, only use small doses in the short term. It can cause constipation and reduced absorption of nutrients in the digestive tract.

Combines well with
Wood avens (see page 44) for gum disease
Pilewort (see page 50) for haemorrhoids (piles)

Try it in oak flower essence
Flower essences were invented by Dr Edward Bach, who felt that each plant had an energy that could have a balancing effect on our emotions. Oak is for people who soldier on despite adversity and never give up even when the situation is hopeless. Oak flower essence is said to help such people to rest, recuperate and find another way.

Gather some oak flowers on a sunny, spring day and float them in a small glass bowl containing 25 ml (1 fl oz) spring water. Leave the bowl near the oak tree in the sunshine for a few hours so that the energy of the flowers can pass into the water. Lift out the flowers with an oak twig or leaf. Pour the water into a 50 ml (2 fl oz) dropper bottle and add 25 ml (1 fl oz) brandy to preserve it. Label and take 4 drops in a glass of water, as required. Flower essences will keep for three years.

Oak

Forager's checklist
* Stately, long-lived tree
* Widely distributed
* Wavy-edged leaves
* Powerful astringent
* Harvest bark in spring
* Use the flowers for flower essence
* Never strip bark from the main trunk
* Up to 25 m (80 ft) high
* Family: Fagaceae

Ranunculus ficaria

Pilewort

lesser celandine

Woodland plants

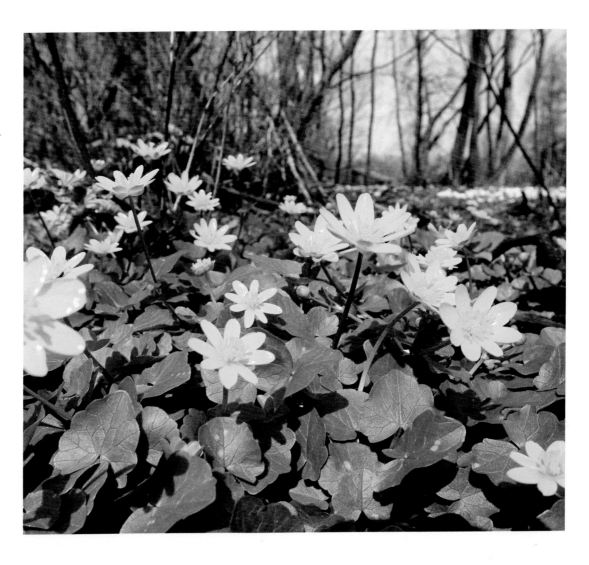

Fact and folklore

Pilewort carpets woodlands with yellow, star-like blooms in early spring. It is a good example of the Doctrine of Signatures – if you carefully uproot a plant, it shows you very clearly what it is used for, as it has little 'piles' on its 'bottom'! It is useful drunk as a dried herb infusion for internal haemorrhoids (piles) and applied externally as a compress for external piles. The tannins are astringent and will help to tone up the blood vessels that are engorged and inflamed causing these irritating little 'bruises' and swellings. Pilewort, when used regularly, can help to relieve the symptoms and reduce attacks.

What to look for

Pilewort grows 5–10 cm (2–4 in) high and 10 cm (4 in) wide. It has a small root system and many small tubers just under the ground from which the leaves and stalk grow. The dark green leaves are kidney-shaped, 2.5 cm (1 in) across. The flowers open in the morning and are closed by sunset. When they are open, they are bright yellow; the underside of the petals is green, however, so when they close they are disguised. Each flower has up to ten petals.

Can be mistaken for

Celandine (*Chelidonium majus*) (see page 134) has a similar common name but is a different plant in both appearance and medicinal properties.

Where to look

Pilewort grows in moist, shady places: woodland, hedgerows, sheltered banks and meadows.

When to look for it

The plant grows from February to May and then dies

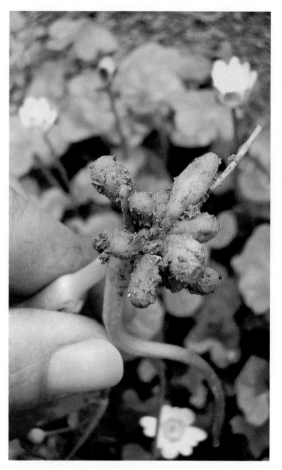

The swollen tubers on the bottom of the pilewort plant are a good example of the Doctrine of Signatures.

back until the following spring.

What to harvest

The whole plant, roots and tops.

What is it good for?

Haemorrhoids (piles)

Pilewort

How to use it

Pick the whole plant, bruise it, allow it to wilt overnight and use it to make pilewort ointment. When dried, the herb may be used as an infusion and drunk. Alternatively, the infusion can be cooled and used as an enema for internal piles.

Cautions

Do not take the fresh herb internally as an infusion. Do not use internally during pregnancy.

Combines well with

Horse chestnut (see page 38) internally and externally for haemorrhoids (piles)
Yarrow (see page 84) and silverweed (see page 70) internally and externally for haemorrhoids (piles)

Try it in pilewort ointment

Infuse some chopped, wilted fresh pilewort in sunflower oil over a bain-marie for two hours. Strain out the herb, replace with fresh herb and infuse again. Combine the resulting oil with 25 ml (1 fl oz) yarrow-infused oil and add 5 g (1/4 oz) beeswax. Melt this in a pan over a low heat and test the setting consistency with a cold teaspoon. If it is not hard enough, add more beeswax until the desired setting consistency is reached. Pour into a jar to set. Label. Use as required topically on irritated piles. It will keep for about a year. If it smells good it is still effective.

Forager's checklist

* **Earliest spring flower**
* **Widely distributed**
* **Piles on its bottom!**
* **Fresh herb used externally**
* **Bright yellow flowers**
* **Astringent**
* **5–10 cm (2–4 in) high and 10 cm (4 in) wide**
* **Family: Ranunculaceae**

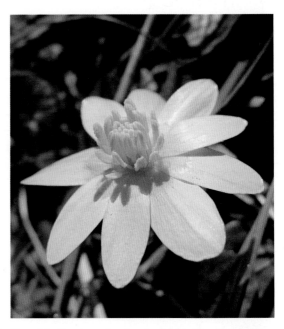

One of the first signs of spring, the bright yellow flowers bring much welcomed colour to the bare earth after the winter.

Scrophularia nodosa

Figwort

knotted figwort

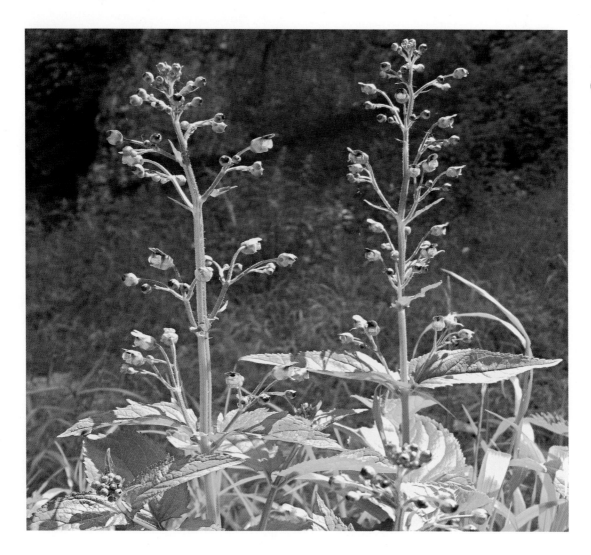

Fact and folklore

Scrophularia derives from the fact that figwort was used to treat scrofula (the traditional name for chronic skin disease) and *nodosa* refers to its knobbly roots. In the past, scrofula was most commonly caused by a type of tuberculosis. Figwort was traditionally used as a poultice for the skin, and herbalists continue to use it for skin disease today. It is a blood cleanser and wound healer.

There is not much modern research about it, and it continues to be used because of its traditional record and because of the experiences of modern herbalists who are able to bear testament to its effectiveness. It works well internally and externally for thickened, itching skin problems such as psoriasis, chronic eczema and dermatitis. It is especially indicated for infections of the skin such as boils and abscesses, and herbalists use it for treating the very infectious condition, impetigo, both as a poultice and taken internally. It also strengthens the beat of the heart.

What to look for

Figwort is a perennial plant that grows up to 1.2 m (4 ft) high and 30 cm (1 ft) wide. Square, branching stems grow from a distinctly knobbly, tuberous root. The leaves are heart-shaped and have roughly serrated edges. The tiny, insignificant flowers, only 3–5 mm ($1/8$–$1/4$ in) across, have two upper and lower lobes. They are a purplish-reddish brown and form towards the top of the stems.

Can be mistaken for

The stems of water figwort (*Scrophularia aquatica*), which grows in close proximity to water, have winged projections; its leaves are not as heart-shaped and they have round, toothed edges. It does not have the

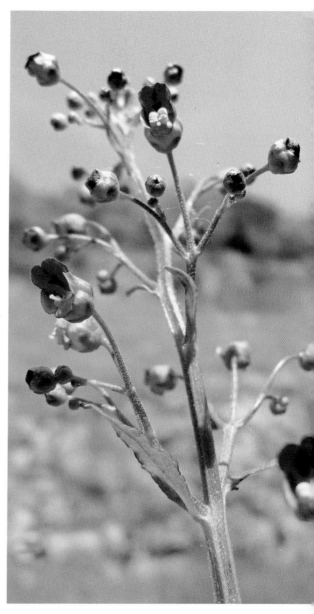

The small, insignificant flowers of figwort are easy to miss but they are much loved by the bees for their nectar.

characteristic knobbly root but a fibrous, branching root system. Water figwort has a traditional reputation as a skin cleansing and healing remedy, but is not used much by modern herbalists.

Where to look
Figwort grows in damp and shaded ground by footpaths, on woodland banks and in damp hedgerows.

When to look for it
Figwort grows from March to September and flowers from July to September.

What to harvest
The whole flowering plant.

What is it good for?
Boils • Psoriasis

How to use it
Pick the fresh leaves, pulverize them and use them as a poultice on scabby, itching skin conditions; to bring boils to a head, bandage on and leave in place for an hour, at least twice a day. Collect the whole herb just as it is coming into flower and dry it, then make a tincture for internal use for chronic skin disease. Discard the tincture after six months. The dose of figwort is much smaller than standard tincture doses, at 0.5 ml (see page 35) up to three times a day. Figwort is a strong herb that has cardiac effects and in large doses may be purgative. It is best used in combination with other lymphatic herbs such as cleavers, blood cleansers such as burdock and liver herbs such as yellow dock. For treating infections, combine it with an anti-infective, immune-boosting herb such as wild garlic.

Forager's checklist
* **Perennial herb**
* **Widely distributed**
* **Lymphatic and skin cleanser**
* **Knobbly root distinguishes from water figwort**
* **Do not use the fresh leaves internally**
* **Harvest the whole plant in flower**
* **Up to 1.2 m (4 ft) high and 30 cm (1 ft) wide**
* **Family: Scrophulariaceae**

Cautions
It increases the strength of heart contractions, so do not use in heart problems, or if palpitations or rapid irregular heartbeats are a problem. Fresh leaves are acrid and cause nausea and vomiting if taken internally, and large doses are purgative. Do not use in pregnancy. It is advised to take this herb with the supervision of a medical herbalist.

Combines well with
Cleavers (see page 172), burdock (see page 125) and yellow dock (see page 108) for psoriasis
Wild garlic (see page 41) for skin infections

Figwort

Tilia spp.

Lime

linden blossom

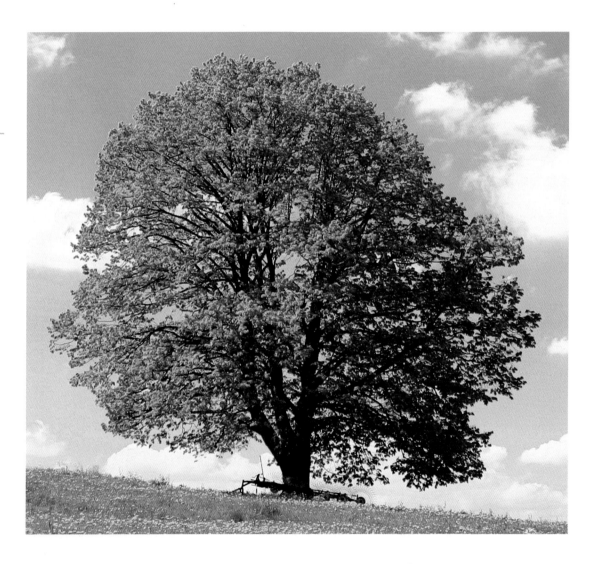

Fact and folklore

This beautiful tree is found throughout Europe. In France, its flowers are used as a popular tisane known as *tilleul*. The scent of the flowers attracts bees and hoverflies, and the sweet heavy smell of the flowers fills the air when you are walking underneath one. Harvesting lime blossom is a slow and relaxing pastime that will bear reward in the form of blissful infusions for the rest of the year.

Lime blossom is a soporific that calms the nerves and relaxes the blood vessels and muscles. It opens the peripheral circulation, lowering the blood pressure and allowing sweating and cooling in fevers. It has been shown to be beneficial for children's infections, speeding recovery and reducing complications. It can be taken for stress and anxiety and to induce a restful night's sleep. It is also rich in flavonoids that have restorative properties on the lining of blood vessels.

What to look for

This large, rounded canopy tree, up to 30 m (100 ft) high, often with a flat underside, is found especially in pastures as livestock graze upon them. It has light green, heart-shaped leaves. The 'flowers' are technically bracts, and have a flat, papery thin, oval-shaped, leaf-like structure from which 4–10 flowers grow on a thin, branching stem. The flowers are 5–10 mm ($^1/_4$–$^1/_2$ in) across, and have five yellow-green sepals and five pale yellow petals, with many stamens in the centre. Broad-leaved lime (*Tilia platyphyllos*), common lime (*T.* x *europaea*) and small-leaved lime (*T. cordata*) are all similar.

Can be mistaken for

The flowering bracts of lime are unmistakable and the various species are, medicinally, largely interchangeable.

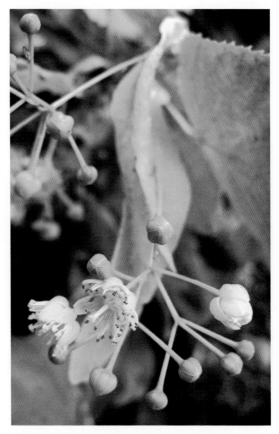

When harvesting limeflowers collect the whole flower; the papery bract, stems and blossoms.

Where to look

Lime trees are found in parks, gardens, woodland and meadows.

When to look for it

It flowers in July.

What to harvest

The whole flowers, bracts and blossoms.

Lime

What is it good for?

Restless leg syndrome • Coughs • Sore throat • Atherosclerosis • Chilblains • High cholesterol • High blood pressure • Varicose veins • Anxiety and stress • Insomnia • Fever

How to use it

Gather the flowers when most of them are just about to open and they are fragrant. Make a fresh herb tincture with the flower blossoms. Dry them for use as a delicately fragrant infusion. The fresh flowers may also be used for infusion. Drink regularly to reduce stress and for high blood pressure as a blood vessel restorative and relaxant. Take hot to induce sweating and restful sleep in fevers. For children, sweeten with a little honey. Take as an infusion in the evening to promote a restful night's sleep.

Cautions

If treating high blood pressure, it is advisable to do so with the assistance of a registered medical herbalist and your doctor.

Combines well with

Elder (see page 184) for fevers, colds and viral illness
Yarrow (see page 84), mistletoe (see page 59) and Hawthorn (see page 166) for high blood pressure
Chamomile (see page 102) and St John's wort (see page 137) for stress, anxiety and insomnia

Try it in infused limeflower honey

This is a beautifully fragrant sweet treat that well preserves all the therapeutic properties of limeflowers. Put fresh flowers into a pan and, pressing them down, just cover them with runny honey. Gently heat on a low setting for an hour. Pour off the honey into a jar, straining out the flowers if preferred. They may remain in, however. Label and take 1 teaspoon as required for stress and anxiety and give to children for feverish colds, coughs and sore throats. Alternatively, use on toast or to sweeten herbal teas as a daily treat for stressful times. Do not give to children under 2 years old (see page 35). This will keep up to six months or more in the refrigerator, if you don't eat it all before then.

Forager's checklist

* **Deciduous tree**
* **Widely distributed**
* **Sweet-scented blossoms**
* **Loved by bees**
* **Flowers in July**
* **Widely cultivated in parks and gardens**
* **Often planted along roads**
* **Relaxing diaphoretic, induces sweating in fevers**
* **Restorative to blood vessels**
* **Also known as linden blossom**
* **30 m (100 ft) high**
* **Family: Tiliaceae**

Viscum album

Mistletoe

birdlime mistletoe

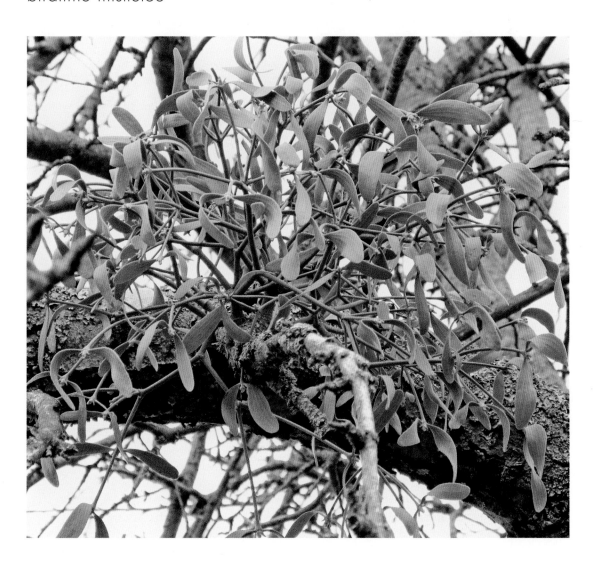

Mistletoe

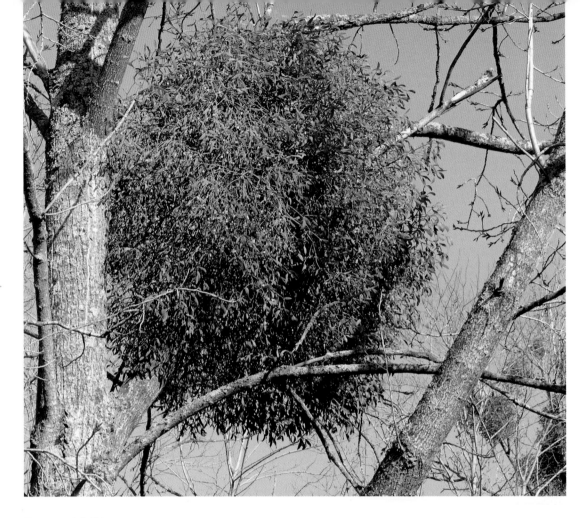

Fact and folklore

Sacred to the Druids as the plant that would heal all ills, tradition states that mistletoe was cut with a golden sickle in an annual ceremony and a sprig was distributed to all the people watching. The Christmas ritual of kissing under the mistletoe still persists today. Birds, especially the mistle thrush, love to eat the berries, which are sticky and become glued to the bird's beak. The bird then wipes its beak clean on the rough bark of a tree where the seed later germinates.

Mistletoe is evergreen but is usually only visible in winter when the trees it lives on are bare.

Mistletoe berries are poisonous, but the leaves and shoots are powerful medicine for the central nervous system. It is used for high blood pressure and palpitations, to relax the blood vessel walls and strengthen and steady the heartbeat. It will relax deep nervous tension in the body and is useful for headaches caused by tight neck muscles and migraines. It also has a reputation for relieving pain from pinched and trapped nerves. Research has shown mistletoe as having anti-tumour effects, meaning it may have a part to play in oncology treatments. Mistletoe also contains high levels of zinc, which may contribute to its positive immune-boosting properties.

What to look for

It forms a compact green ball, 30–150 cm (1–5 ft) in diameter, and is especially visible in trees during winter. Mistletoe has many-branching, thick stems each ending in a greenish-yellow, paired, oval leaf structure with parallel veins. Insignificant yellow flowers are followed by the recognizable translucent, white berries.

Can be mistaken for

What is called mistletoe in the USA is *Phoradendron serotinum* and is no relation. It is poisonous.

Where to look

Mistletoe is a parasitic plant and most commonly grows in old apple orchards but is also found growing in oak, ash, hawthorn, lime and larch trees.

When to look for it

In deciduous trees, from November to April when the trees have no leaves and the green ball of mistletoe is easily visible.

What to harvest

The stems and leaves.

What is it good for?

High blood pressure • Headache • Migraine

How to use it

Remove and discard any berries, then dry the herb for use in cold water infusions for high blood pressure and nervous tension. Make a tincture for combination with other herb tinctures and for use as a smaller than standard dose of 0.5–1 ml (see page 35) for headache, blood pressure and compressed nerve pain.

Cautions

Although research shows that mistletoe is of value in the treatment of cancer, it must only be used with the assistance of an oncologist and a medical herbalist. The berries are poisonous; always remove them from the plant before preparing. Do not use in pregnancy. Treatment of high blood pressure and general use should be under supervision of a medical herbalist.

Combines well with

Cramp bark (see page 187) and hawthorn (see page 166) for high blood pressure

Forager's checklist

❋ **Parasitic upon trees**

❋ **Widely distributed**

❋ **Easily seen in midwinter**

❋ **Nervous system relaxant**

❋ **Harvest the leaves and small stems in winter**

❋ **Berries are poisonous**

❋ **Plants spread in the main by birds**

❋ **30–150 cm (1–5 ft) across**

❋ **Family: Viscaceae**

Mistletoe

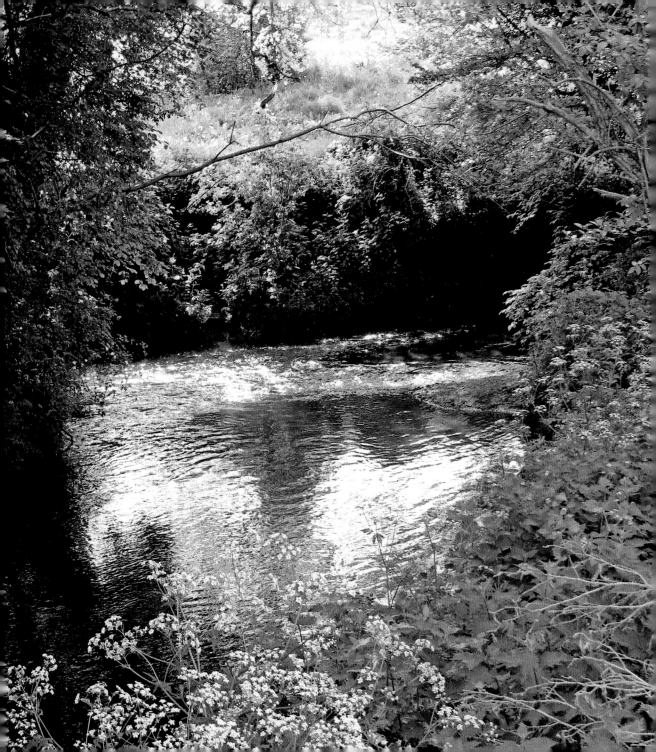

RIVERSIDE PLANTS

Waterways such as rivers, streams and canals, as well as lakes, ponds and marshes, are invariably a delight to behold. Watching the water slip away with such ease and grace makes this one of the most pleasurable environments in which to forage. The sound of a babbling brook is music to harvest to and the lush greenness of the plants that the moist soil attracts, holds a multitude of healing properties just waiting to be discovered.

Althaea officinalis/Malva sylvestris

Mallow

marsh mallow, common mallow

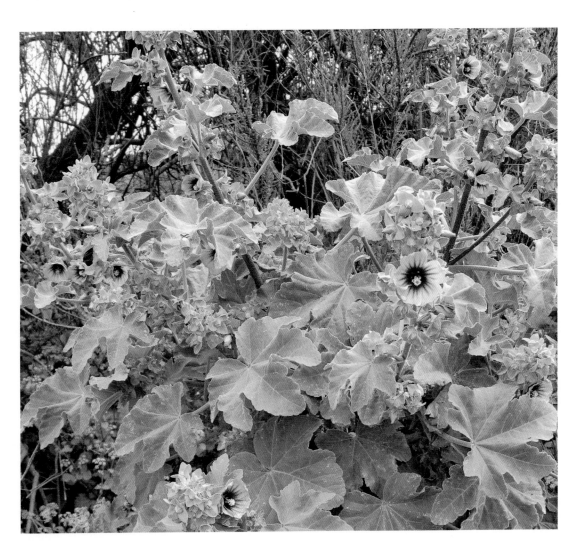

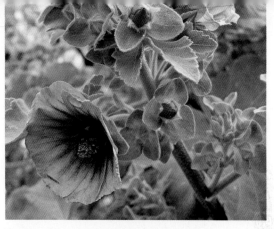

The beautiful, pink flowers of the common mallow (*Malva sylvestris*) impart their colour into syrups.

Fact and folklore

Plants in the genera *Althaea* and *Malva* all contain large quantities of a sticky substance called mucilage. The name *Althaea* comes from the Greek *altho* meaning 'to cure'. Mallows have been used as food and medicine since Egyptian times, and the roots are quite palatable if boiled then fried with butter and garlic. They were widely cultivated in country gardens for their healing and nutritious qualities.

Mucilage is useful for conditions where the tissues are hot and inflamed, by providing a soothing 'plaster' over the top. Internally, they have an effect from the mouth right through the digestive tract, and also in the lungs and the urinary tract by reflex action. They can be used topically for dry, irritated skin conditions and also as drawing poultices for splinters and boils.

What to look for

Marsh mallow (*Althaea officinalis*) is a perennial herb rising each spring from a thick, spreading root system into a tall, branching plant, 1–1.2 m (3–4 ft) high and 1 m (3 ft) wide. The flowers are 2–12 cm (1–5 in) across and vary from light to deep pink through to lilac, and have five petals. The central calyx protrudes; the colour varies between species, being usually pink or yellow. The seeds develop in round, cheese-shaped pods. Mallow (*Malva sylvestris*) is a perennial herb that readily selfseeds, growing in a similar habit to marsh mallow. The leaves are round with 5–7 lobes and covered with a fine down. The flowers are pink with dark pink veins and calyx. They have five notched petals. The seeds are similar to those of marsh mallow.

Can be mistaken for

All plants that belong in the Malvaceae family are interchangeable medicinally.

Where to look

They are found all over Europe, much cultivated but also growing in the wild on waste ground, footpaths, meadows and moist ground. Marsh mallow itself is found in marshes near the sea.

When to look for it

They all grow from April to November, flowering from June to August.

What to harvest

The leaves, roots and flowers.

What is it good for?

Acne rosacea • Boils • Asthma • Bronchitis • Coughs • Sore throat • Diarrhoea • Heartburn • Indigestion • Cystitis • Kidney stones

How to use it

Use the fresh or dried leaves in cold infusions (the mucilage is largely destroyed by hot water) to drink for treatment of inflammation of the digestive, respiratory and urinary tracts. Leave it to infuse over night in cold water. Make a fresh herb tincture, which

Mallow

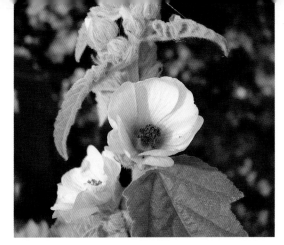

The delicate pink flower of marsh mallow (*Althaea officinalis*) may be used for a soothing syrup.

extracts the mucilage. Harvest the root in autumn when it contains the highest concentration of mucilage. Make a fresh root tincture with it or dry it for use in cold maceration. Pulverize a fresh leaf or piece of root as a poultice, holding it in place with a dressing or plaster. Change every 12 hours. Moistened dried leaf or root can be used in the same way. Make a syrup from the flowers or leaves for dry coughs and sore throats.

Cautions
Any unexplained bleeding from the bladder or bowel should be investigated by your doctor. Bleeding from the upper digestive tract presents as thick, tarry, black stools.

Combines well with
Meadowsweet (see page 169) and chamomile (see page 102) for gastritis and heartburn
Couch grass (see page 90) and plantain (see page 105) for urinary infection

Try it in pink flower syrup
For treating dry coughs and sore throats, gather mallow flowers on a dry day. Put them in a pan and just cover them with water. Simmer gently for 15 minutes. Strain and reserve the liquid and repeat using this liquid with fresh flowers. Strain and return the liquid to the pan. Simmer and reduce the liquid by a third. Measure the resulting liquid. For every 200 ml (7 fl oz) of liquid, add 400 ml (14 fl oz) honey or 150 g (5 oz) sugar. Stir over a low heat, until dissolved, then bring to the boil for five minutes. Bottle and store in the refrigerator for up to six months.
Doses are:
- Under 5 years: 1 teaspoon
- 5–10 years: 1–2 teaspoons
- Over 10 years: 1 dessertspoon

Forager's checklist
- ✳ **Perennial herbaceous shrub**
- ✳ **Common garden visitor**
- ✳ ***Malva* and *Althaea* have similar properties**
- ✳ **Roots contain more mucilage in autumn**
- ✳ **Harvest leaves, roots and flowers**
- ✳ **Soothing tonic for the mucous membrane**
- ✳ **1–1.2 m (3–4 ft) high and 1 m (3 ft) wide**
- ✳ **Family: Malvaceae**

Equisetum arvense

Horsetail

field horsetail, pewterwort, bottlebrush

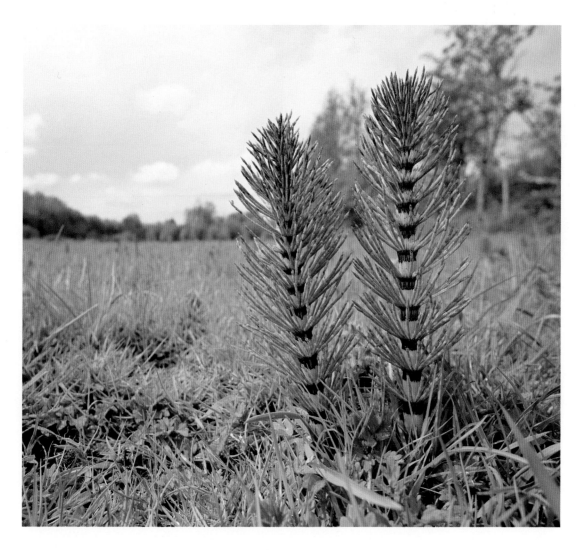

Fact and folklore

The horsetails are closely allied to the ferns and are considered to be ancient plants; there are fossilized remains of giant horsetail specimens. The Latin word *equus* means 'horse' and *seta* means 'bristle'. It is also called pewterwort and bottlebrush because it was used as a scouring brush on pewter and kitchen implements. Tradition has it that horsetails growing indicate underground water.

The Doctrine of Signatures implies its use for joint problems because of its jointed growing habit. This is confirmed by the fact that it is rich in the mineral silica, which is essential for the connective tissue repair of ligaments, tendons and bones. Silica is also essential for strong hair and nails. Horsetail is also rich in iron, potassium, manganese, magnesium, chromium and vitamin A. It is most commonly used as a mineral restorative for osteoporosis and broken bones. Horsetail has restorative effects on the structures of the urinary system and is used for urinary symptoms such as prostate problems, cystitis, bedwetting and the passing of stones. Its tannins are also astringent and help to tone the membranes of the urinary system, reducing bleeding and increasing resistance to invasion by infective organisms.

What to look for

Fruiting stems grow in early spring, from a deep and wide root system, up to 60 cm (2 ft) high. They are short and stout with a cone-like top from which spores are shed. These stems then die back and sterile stems appear. These consist of sections with serrated edges around their circumference. The plant gradually branches into progressively narrower stems, all sectioned at roughly 2.5 cm (1 in) intervals. The plant becomes increasingly brittle as it gets older. Horsetails

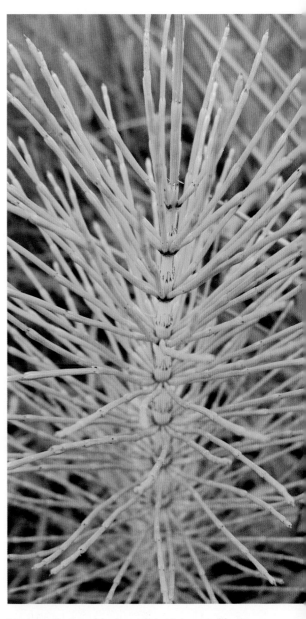

It is the sterile stem of the horsetail that is harvested for its medicinal properties.

are often found growing en masse and are difficult to eradicate from gardens.

Can be mistaken for
Related plants such as *Equisetum sylvaticum*, *E. maximum* and *E. hyemale* may also be used. Other horsetail varieties.

Where to look
It is found mostly in wet ground by steams, springs and boggy ditches.

When to look for it
The fruiting stems grow in April and the sterile stems grow from May to October.

What to harvest
The whole sterile plant stems – best harvested early in the season before they become tough and brittle.

What is it good for?
Arthritis • Osteoporosis • Cystitis • Incontinence • Kidney stones • Prostate problems

How to use it
Pick the young fresh stems and use fresh or dry as an infusion for urinary infections. The dried, powdered herb can be put into capsules to provide essential minerals to be taken regularly for joint and bone disease. The fresh herb tincture preserves its properties well, including the silica. Juice the fresh herb and store by freezing in ice-cube trays, taking one defrosted cube up to twice a day. Alternatively, preserve with alcohol by adding 50 ml (2 fl oz) alcohol for every 50 ml (2 fl oz) juice. Take 1 dessertspoon up to twice a day, either neat or diluted in water.

Forager's checklist
* **Persistent perennial weed**
* **Widely distributed**
* **Jointed stems**
* **Source of silica**
* **Pick sterile stems when young**
* **60 cm (2 ft) high**
* **Family: Equisetaceae**

Cautions
Some people may find this herb harsh on the lining of an inflamed bladder, so combine with plantain, mallow or comfrey.

Combines well with
Nettle (see page 155) for osteoporosis
Plantain (see page 105) and shepherd's purse (see page 131) for blood in the urine

Try it in horsetail juice
Difficult to extract, but worth the effort. Horsetail needs to be juiced in a heavy-duty juicer. Hand juicers will only yield small quantities of juice before they break under the pressure of tough horsetail stems. Collect a large quantity of soft horsetail stems and press them through the juicer. Preserve the juice with as high proof alcohol as possible (50 per cent). Use 2 parts juice to 1 part alcohol. The juice will keep in the refrigerator for one month. Take 1 dessertspoon twice a day for prostate and bladder problems and also for joint repair.

Horsetail

Potentilla anserina
Silverweed
prince's feathers

Fact and folklore

It is called silverweed because of its attractive, pale, silvery foliage that resembles the feathers on the Prince of Wales' crest. It has been recently renamed *Argentina anserina* because 'argent' means silver. Silverweed is rich in tannins and is used as an astringent herb for bleeding of the gums, digestive tract and haemorrhoids (piles). It is also used for blood in the urine from bladder irritation or infection and in cases of excessive menstrual bleeding. It can be injected into the nostrils for nosebleeds or given as an enema for internal bleeding piles. It is also effective for diarrhoea, to tone up the bowels. The tannins will also tone up the mucous membranes of the throat, so it can be used as a gargle for sore throats.

What to look for

Silverweed is a low-growing perennial plant with attractive foliage, which appears silvery because of the fine, white, silky hairs that cover the leaves. It grows 15–25 cm (6–10 in) tall and 15–25 cm (6–10 in) wide. Many opposite-paired leaves are interspersed by small leaflets. The leaf edges are finely cut. Single yellow flowers, each with five petals with many stamens in the centre, are borne at the top of short stems.

Can be mistaken for

Both tormentil (*Potentilla erecta*) and creeping cinquefoil (*P. reptans*) also have deeply cut leaves with similar yellow flowers, although tormentil often only has four petals. Both plants have similar properties to silverweed.

Where to look

It is commonly found in damp, sandy soils in close proximity to water.

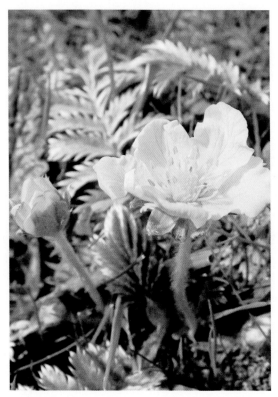

Identification of silverweed, despite its buttercup-like flowers, is easily confirmed by its silvery-grey foliage.

When to look for it

From March to November, it flowers in June and July.

What to harvest

The whole herb.

What is it good for?

Gums and teeth • Mouth ulcers • Sore throat • Bleeding • Haemorrhoids (piles) • Nosebleed • Diarrhoea • Irritable bowel syndrome • Cystitis • Heavy periods

Silverweed

How to use it

Harvest the herb just before it flowers and dry it for use in infusions for diarrhoea, and as mouthwashes and gargles for gum disease and sore throats. Use the infusion as a compress or enema for bleeding haemorrhoids (piles), or as nosedrops for nosebleeds. Make a fresh or dry herb tincture for internal use and to include in cream for piles.

Cautions

Do not treat acute infected diarrhoea with astringent herbs as it is the body's way of flushing the infective organisms out of the body. Do not use tannin-rich herbs for long periods internally.

Combines well with

Wood avens (see page 44) for gum disease
Nettle (see page 155) and shepherd's purse (see page 131) for heavy periods

Try it in silverweed sore throat gargle

This infusion is of benefit for the treatment of enlarged tonsils and sore throats. Infuse 25 g (1 oz) of dried, or 50 g (2 oz) of fresh silverweed leaves in 300 ml (1/2 pint) boiling water. Leave for at least 20 minutes before straining. Gargle with 50 ml (2 fl oz) of the infusion for a minute every two hours for acute sore throats, or three times a day for chronically enlarged tonsils.

Forager's checklist

* **Perennial herb**
* **Widely distributed**
* **Distinct silvery foliage**
* **Astringent**
* **Use the whole herb**
* **Harvest before flowering**
* **15–25 cm (6–10 in) tall and 15–25 cm (6–10 in) wide**
* **Family: Rosaceae**

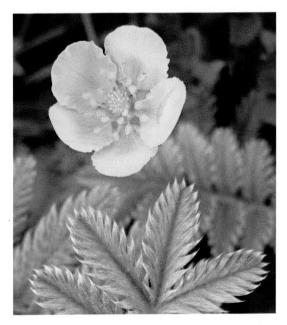

Chew a piece of fresh leaf to experience the astringent and drying effects of the tannins in silverweed.

Salix spp.

Willow

white willow, european willow, crack willow, grey willow

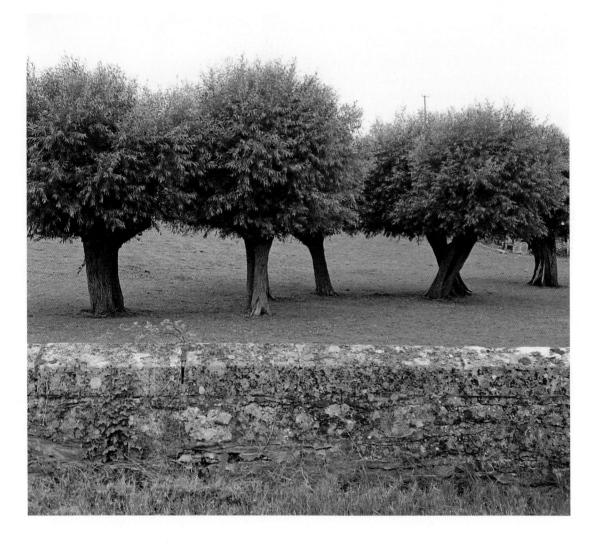

Fact and folklore

The name *Salix* comes from the Celtic *sal* meaning 'near to' and *lis* meaning 'water'. There are many species of willow, the white or European willow (*S. alba*) being the most commonly written about medicinally. Crack willow (*S. fragilis*), grey willow (*S. cinerea*) and purple willow (*S. purpurea*) are also used medicinally. The root bark of the American black willow (*S. nigra*) is used medicinally, but has different properties, mainly being used as an anaphrodisiac.

Records of the medicinal uses of willow exist from 4,000 years ago and throughout history. It is famous for being the source of salicin, which was first isolated and extracted by a French chemist in the early 1800s. Salicin is converted to salicylic acid, which is from where the non-steroidal, anti-inflammatory drug aspirin was formulated. Salicylic acid is caustic on the lining of the stomach, causing irritation and bleeding. When used in the form of willow bark, the other constituents buffer these irritating effects and provide some protection to the stomach membranes. Willow bark is used for anti-inflammatory effects, which it achieves by inhibiting and stimulating production of various different inflammatory and anti-inflammatory substances called prostaglandins in the body. This is useful for treatment of joint and muscle aches as felt in arthritis, polymyalgia and feverish infections.

What to look for

Willows are large deciduous trees, to 25 m (80 ft) high, with thick, fissured bark on old trunks and branches and whip-like, yellowy-green new stems that grow vigorously every spring. The long, thin leaves are dark green on the upper side and pale underneath. The trees bear either male or female flowers, before the leaves in the early spring, in the form of catkins.

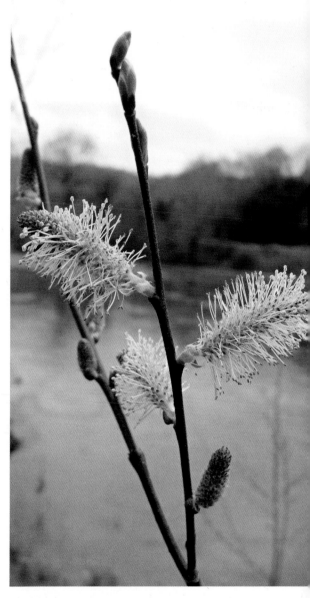

A male willow flower in the early spring – both female and male flowers emerge before the leaves.

The seeds emerge in June on a fine, silky fluff that floats easily on the slightest breeze.

Can be mistaken for
Other species of willow.

Where to look
Willows thrive in damp ground, by rivers, lakes and marshes. They regenerate rapidly after being cut back.

When to look for it
The catkins appear in March, the leaves in April and the seeds in early June – usually seen as a fine, wind-borne down.

What to harvest
The bark.

What is it good for?
Arthritis • Gout • Fever

How to use it
It is easiest to strip the bark from 2–3-year-old branches and shoots and dry it for use in a decoction or to make a fresh bark tincture. Take either of these internally for their anti-inflammatory effects.

Cautions
Avoid if taking aspirin or other non-steroidal, anti-inflammatory medication and with gastritis or ulceration of the digestive tract or blood clotting disorders.

Combines well with
Nettle (see page 155) and dandelion root (see page 114) for inflammatory joint and muscle conditions, arthritis and gout

Forager's checklist

* ❋ **Fast-growing tree**
* ❋ **Widely distributed**
* ❋ **Long, narrow leaves**
* ❋ **Common waterside and wet-ground tree**
* ❋ **Stems will root and grow easily when stuck in the ground**
* ❋ **Look for prunings and windfall branches of young trees**
* ❋ **Source of salicin**
* ❋ **25 m (80 ft) high**
* ❋ **Family: Salicaceae**

Willow

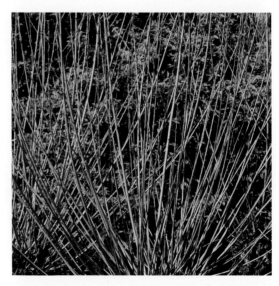

Coppiced willow is an excellent sustainable source of willow bark that rapidly regenerates after harvesting.

Symphytum officinalis

Comfrey

knitbone

Riverside plants

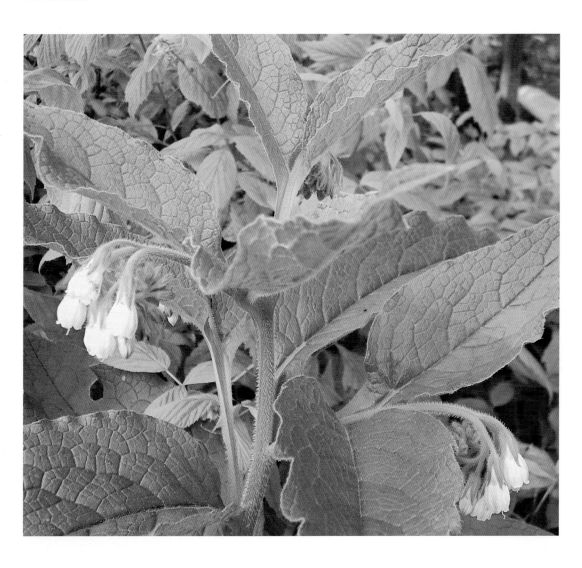

Fact and folklore

Comfrey's names refer to its ability to repair tissues: bone and flesh. Comfrey comes from the Latin *con firma* and *Symphytum* from the Greek *symphylos*, meaning 'to unite'. It has been used since ancient times for its wound-healing powers and continues to be used by herbalists today. There are also records of it having been eaten as a spring vegetable.

Comfrey has been scrutinized over the last few years because it contains potentially liver-damaging compounds called pyrollizidine alkaloids. However, examination of records of herbalists who have used it internally over the last hundred years have not flagged up any problems and scrutiny of modern reports fail to provide clear conclusions. It is left to the discretion of individual herbalists whether they use comfrey leaf internally, but it is recommended for short-term use only, a few weeks at the most. The root is for external use only.

The rapid healing that it brings about can be seen very quickly. Allantoin is the substance responsible and it has been shown to penetrate deep into the tissues. It is used for ulcers throughout the digestive tract and topically for ulcerations and wounds of the skin. It will also speed the repair of muscle, ligament and tendon injuries, and if applied over broken bones can speed the 'knitting' of the edges together.

What to look for

Comfrey is a perennial plant that grows 60–120 cm (2–4 ft) high and 60 cm (2 ft) wide. It grows each spring from a thick, white root that is extremely slimy inside. The large oval leaves, with a pointed tip, emerge in a clump from the base. The whole plant is covered with short, rough, bristly hairs. The flower stems have leaves growing partway up them, and the

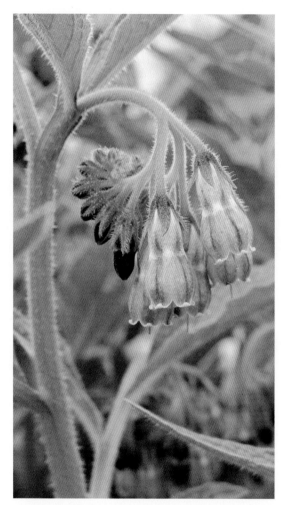

The wound-healing substance, allantoin is concentrated in the flowering tops of comfrey.

flowers form in a curled stalk at the top. The flowers are small, 3–5 mm ($1/8$–$1/4$ in) across, and bell-shaped with a green calyx. They are usually a pale yellow-cream, but there are many variations in colour from pink through to blue.

Comfrey

Can be mistaken for

There are different varieties of comfrey that are all interchangeable medicinally. However, it is thought that Russian comfrey (*Symphytum* x *uplandicum*) contains higher quantities of pyrollizidine alkaloids. The early spring leaves may resemble foxgloves, but foxglove leaves form a more definite rosette and are covered with soft, downy hairs.

Where to look

Comfrey thrives in damp ground and in partial shade, by rivers and on shady hedge banks. It is often cultivated by gardeners as it makes excellent plant food and compost. It is difficult to eradicate.

When to look for it

The leaves start to grow in March and the plant flowers from June to July. Harvest the root in autumn or early spring.

What to harvest

Flowering tops and the root.

What is it good for?

Bruises • Burns • Psoriasis • Wounds • Arthritis • Backache • Osteoporosis • Sprains and strains • Varicose veins (varicose eczema) • Heartburn • Dry skin conditions

How to use it

Make the tops or root into an infused oil and use as an ointment base to heal all bumps, bruises and cuts. The root is decidedly more mucilaginous than the tops and may be more effective for using on dry, scaly skin as seen around varicose ulcers and in varicose eczema. The fresh herb or root can also be pulverized and used as a poultice for severe contusions, sprains and strains; change it every four hours. Make a tincture of the fresh herb and take internally for the healing of gastric, duodenal and large bowel ulcers (see 'Cautions' below).

Cautions

Be informed about comfrey's content of potential liver-damaging compounds before you decide to take it internally. If you choose to do so, it is recommended for only a few weeks' use. Do not use internally during pregnancy or for children. Do not use comfrey on deep wounds, as it may heal over the top leaving a cavity underneath.

Combines well with

Meadowsweet (see page 169) and chamomile (see page 102) for gastric irritation and ulcers
Plantain (see page 105) and chamomile (see page 102) for ulcerated bowel

Forager's checklist

❋ **Perennial herb**

❋ **Widely distributed**

❋ **Large, rough leaves**

❋ **Harvest roots in autumn or early spring**

❋ **Harvest the flowering tops**

❋ **Wound healer**

❋ **60–120 cm (2–4 ft) high and 60 cm (2 ft) wide**

❋ **Family: Boraginaceae**

Valeriana officinalis

Valerian

all heal

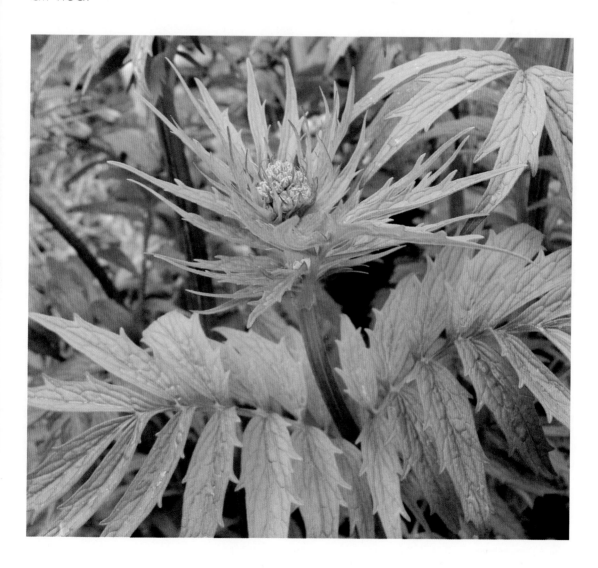

Fact and folklore

The flowers have a strong, heady perfume and the root an earthy, heavy scent that cats adore. During medieval times, it was held in great esteem and was called 'all heal'. It is said that the drug valium was named after this plant, as they have similar properties. Valerian is a wonderful sedative and powerful relaxant without the addictive elements seen with valium use. It can be used to relax tension throughout the body, from pain and spasm in muscles or organs. If an over-active mind is causing anxiety and nervousness, it will induce a relaxed feeling and help to give a good night's sleep. It is of value in reducing symptoms of drug withdrawal, especially benzodiazepines and opiates. Occasionally some people are very sensitive to valerian and it may agitate them, causing wakefulness and anxiety. See 'Cautions' for further information.

What to look for

Valerian is a perennial with a shallow root system that has a pungent scent. The leaves are green with a purple hue when just emerging, and they have serrated edges. The flowering stem is 60–120 cm (2–4 ft) tall, ridged and hollow. It has some smaller leaves towards the bottom. The top is branched with clusters of small, perfumed, pinky-white flowers.

Can be mistaken for

Red valerian (*Centranthus ruber*) is a garden escape that often grows in rocky walls. It has rose-red flowers and oval leaves.

Where to look

Valerian favours damp and shady ground beside canals and rivers, and in ditches. It is easily cultivated and makes an attractive garden plant.

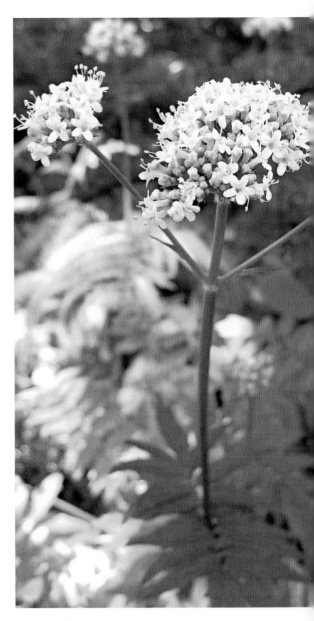

The scent of valerian flowers is highly perfumed and it attracts many pollinating insects.

When to look for it

The leaves begin to grow in April and the flowers appear in July.

What to harvest

The root in autumn or early spring.

What is it good for?

Backache • Cramp • Restless leg syndrome • High blood pressure • Anxiety and stress • Headache • Insomnia • Migraine • Colic • Irritable bowel syndrome (IBS) • Painful periods

How to use it

Make a fresh root tincture. The dried root can be infused (decocting it reduces its effectiveness). Take the tincture instead if the infusion is unpalatable – it has an unusual scent and taste. Use for all types of tissue tension to relax and ease tense muscles and nerves.

Cautions

It has been said that taking valerian may be habit-forming. This depends on the user. It is a better habit than chronic insomnia, panic attacks or a dependence on sleeping pills. It does not have any associated drowsy or hangover effects. Acutely anxious patients should start taking valerian by sipping very small drop doses, as its sedative and relaxing effect may make the body have a counter-reaction and 'jump' into an increased state of alertness. It is advised to treat high blood pressure with the supervision of a medical herbalist.

Combines well with

Chamomile (see page 102) and hop (see page 178) for insomnia and irritable bowel syndrome (IBS)
Wood betony (see page 111) for migraine

Forager's checklist

❋ **Self-seeding perennial**
❋ **Perfumed flowers and scented root**
❋ **Strong relaxant**
❋ **Root is used**
❋ **Harvest in autumn or early spring**
❋ **60–120 cm (2–4 ft) high and 30 cm (1 ft) wide**
❋ **Family: Valerianaceae**

Cats and valerian

If you have a cat, keep your dried valerian where they cannot get it. They love the scent and it is like a drug for them, much like catnip. They will tear open bags to get at it; it also makes them drool and act drunkenly.

Valerian is easily cultivated and readily self-seeds providing new plants for future harvesting.

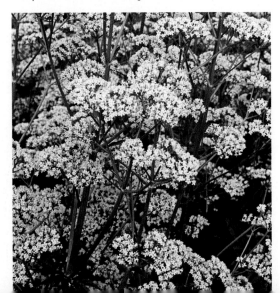

Valerian

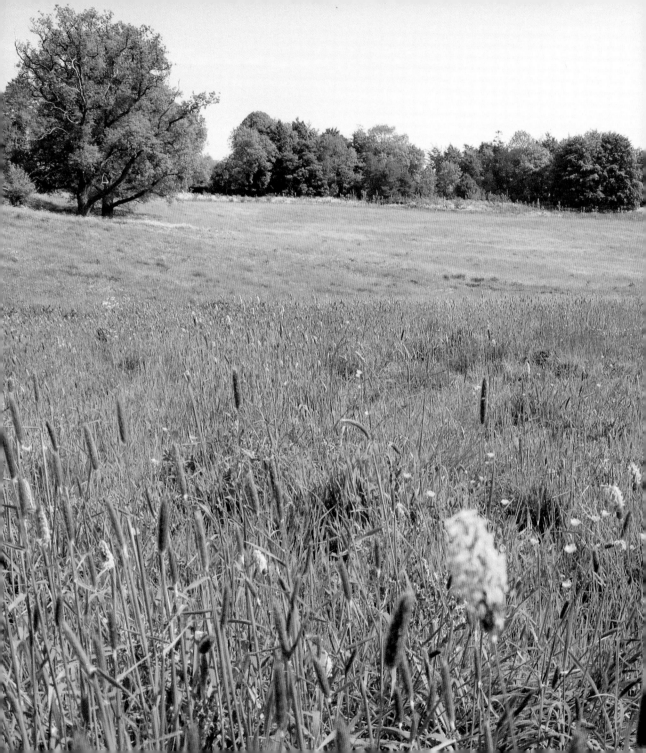

GRASSLAND PLANTS

Grassland and meadows create a wonderful sense of open space. Grasses have their own whispering songs and can resemble the roll of an ocean wave when rippled by a breeze. Some of the plants that inhabit grasslands are considered to be weeds when they come into our gardens, but in the wild they are an integral part of the landscape. Spend some time harvesting from meadows and heaths and you will discover among the microcosm of wildlife all you need for healing.

Achillea millefolium

Yarrow

soldier's woundwort, knight's milfoil

Grassland plants

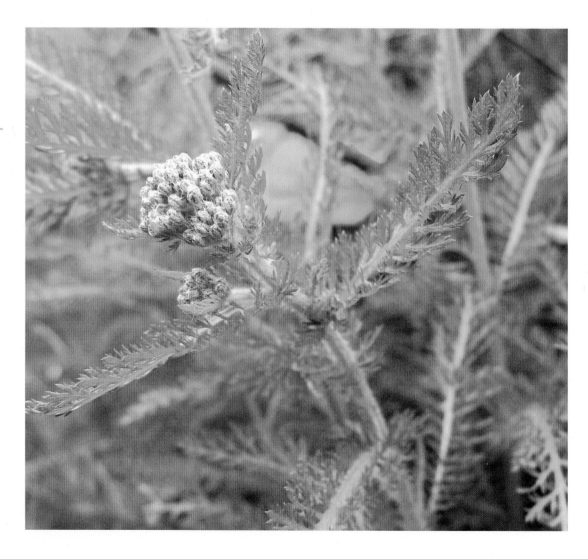

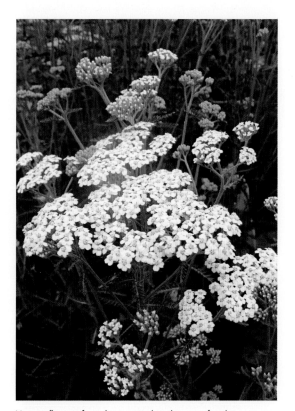

Yarrow

Fact and folklore

This herb was used by Achilles on the battlefield to staunch the flow of blood from the wounds of his soldiers, hence the name *Achillea*; *millefolium* means 'thousand leaves', alluding to its feathery leaf structure. The dried stalks are used in divination in the Chinese system *I Ching*. A maiden who put the herb under her pillow and repeated the following rhyme would dream of her future husband:

'Thou pretty herb of Venus tree, Thy true name is Yarrow, Now who my bosom friend must be, Pray tell thou me tomorrow.'

Yarrow is rich in aromatic and volatile oils that have anti-inflammatory properties similar to those found in chamomile. The herb will stop bleeding from cuts and nosebleeds. If taken internally, it relaxes the muscles surrounding the blood vessels and relieves congested blood flow making it good for period pains, high blood pressure, varicosities and fevers. It has seemingly opposing effects, being good for both bleeding and clotting conditions. It also stimulates the digestion.

What to look for

Feathery, pinnate leaves arise from the base of the plant. The tough, angular stem branches at the top into dense clusters of tiny, yellowish-white flowers. The whole plant is aromatic and grows 30–60 cm (1–2 ft) high.

Can be mistaken for

The leaves and scent of yarrow make this plant quite unmistakable. For this reason, it is difficult to confuse this plant with another, although it has a vague resemblance to wild carrot (*Daucus carota*) which can be differentiated by the pink flower in the centre of its flowerhead.

Yarrow flowers for a long period and it can often be harvested well into September.

Where to look

Yarrow thrives in well-drained soil in most places, especially hedgerows, meadows, waste ground and waysides.

When to look for it

It flowers from June to September. The flowers are long-lived.

What to harvest

The whole flowering plant. Cut through the stems.

What is it good for?

Bites and stings • Bruises • Burns • Cold sores • Eczema • Gums and teeth • Mouth ulcers • Wounds • Colds • Earache • Flu • Sore throat • Bleeding • Chilblains • Haemorrhoids (piles) • High blood pressure • Nosebleed • Varicose veins (for varicose eczema) • Chickenpox and shingles • Fever • Cystitis • Heavy periods • Painful periods

How to use it

The juice of the fresh plant is an excellent first aid herb to stop bleeding and even nosebleeds and also for relieving bites and stings. Cut the plant when it is in flower and make a fresh herb tincture or dry it in small bunches for use as an infusion. The hot infusion will induce sweating to promote natural cooling of a fever in colds and infections or to relieve pain from a period that is slow to start. An infusion makes use of its diuretic, anti-inflammatory and antibacterial effects in the treatment of cystitis. Make an infused oil of the herb to apply topically for wounds and skin rashes. The dried herb may also be used as an infusion in the bath for eczema. The infusion could be used as a cold compress topically for relief of bleeding and inflammation of haemorrhoids (piles), and it is also worth using internally for its ability to 'shunt' stagnant blood around the pelvis. The tincture is used in the treatment of high blood pressure. When its bitterness is unpalatable, a strong root infusion may be used as a mouthwash for toothache and gum disease.

Cautions

Do not use in pregnancy. It may cause skin irritation in people with sensitivity to the daisy family (Compositae). It is advised to treat high blood pressure with the supervision of a medical herbalist.

Forager's checklist

- **Perennial herb**
- **Widely distributed**
- **Avoid if sensitive to daisy family (Compositae)**
- **Harvest whole plant in full flower**
- **Feathery leaves**
- **Aromatic circulatory tonic**
- **30–60 cm (1–2 ft) high**
- **Family: Compositae**

Combines well with

Elderflower (see page 184) and mint (see page 198) in colds, fevers and infection

Couch grass (see page 90) and wild thyme (see page 204) in urinary infection

Mistletoe (see page 59), hawthorn (see page 166) and lime (see page 56) in high blood pressure

Try it in yarrow wound salve

Make an infused oil of yarrow by placing yarrow flowers in a bain-marie and covering them with sunflower oil, then heating gently for two hours. Strain the herb out and replace with fresh flowers, then using the same oil, heat for a further two hours. Strain and add 5 g (1/4 oz) beeswax to 25 ml (1 fl oz) of the oil and heat gently until it melts. Check the setting consistency by dipping in a cold spoon. Add more beeswax if a harder salve is required. Pour into a jar and label. The salve will keep for up to a year. Use on skin irritations to promote healing.

Agrimonia eupatoria

Agrimony

cocklebur

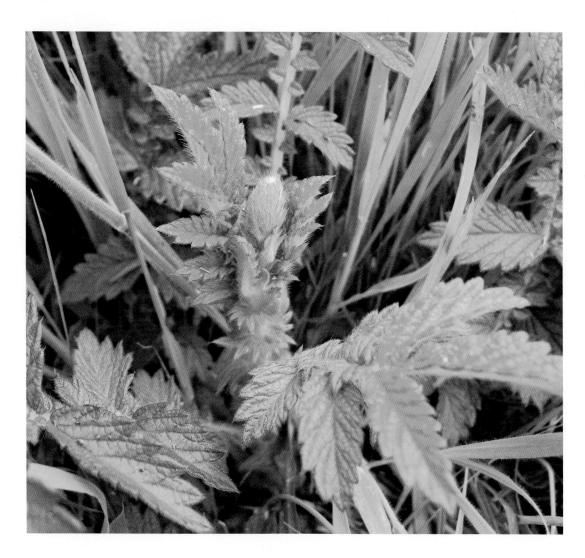

Fact and folklore

The name cocklebur comes from its clingy seeds that hook onto clothing or fur. It was traditionally used as medicine and as a dye plant, and was considered to have powerful magical powers. A medieval rhyme about it states:

'If it be leyd under mann's head,
He shal sleepyn as he were deed;
He shal never drede ne wakyn.
Till fro under his head it be taken.'

Agrimony is a bitter herb that increases bile flow, which is useful in treating gallstones and to improve bowel health. The tannins help to astringe the bowel wall, reducing swelling and inflammation. It has been shown to inhibit the growth of mycobacterium tuberculosis, which may indicate its beneficial effects in helping to normalize gut flora, as does improving digestive function via the liver and improving tone in the bowel wall by making it a less hospitable environment for undesirable flora. It is used for irritable bowel syndrome and inflammatory bowel disease. It will also heal the gut wall, which is useful in chronic inflammatory rheumatic disease where digestive disturbance and a 'leaky gut' is often at the root of the problem. An essence made from the flowers is indicated for people who hide their suffering behind a cheerful façade.

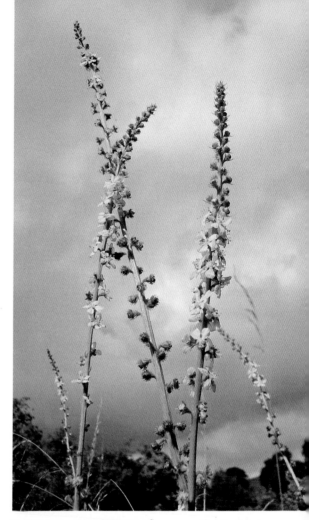

The towering spires of agrimony flowers are often the first sign of their presence in meadows and grassland.

What to look for

Agrimony towers above the other meadow plants, up to 1 m (3 ft) high. The spear-shaped leaves are green on top and silvery-green underneath, covered with fine hairs and with finely serrated edges. It has a round stem and the leaves grow in opposite pairs with small leaflets in between. The flowers are yellow with five petals and grow directly on the tall stem.

The hooked, cone-shaped seeds and the flowers are often seen on the stem at the same time.

Can be mistaken for

Wood avens (see page 44) has a similar leaf and flower structure, but it does not have the same flowering stalk.

Where to look

Agrimony is found growing in grass on sloping meadows and on waste ground.

When to look for it

It grows from May to October and flowers from July to September.

What to harvest

The whole flowering plant.

What is it good for?

Diarrhoea • Diverticular disease • Gallstones • Irritable bowel syndrome (IBS)

How to use it

Collect the whole herb just as it is flowering and make fresh herb tincture. It may be dried for use in infusions. Take it for conditions such as diverticular disease and irritable bowel syndrome (IBS), and for inflammatory bowel diseases like ulcerative colitis and Crohn's disease. Drink the infusion regularly for rheumatoid arthritis with digestive disturbance. Take the infusion every few hours for acute infective diarrhoea and acute diverticular disease. Use the fresh herb tincture as a simple treatment (not in combination with other herbs) for the same conditions or in combination with other herbs for the symptoms of gallstones.

Cautions

None.

Combines well with

Plantain (see page 105) and chamomile (see page 102) for inflammatory bowel conditions

Plantain (see page 105) and hop (see page 178) for diverticular disease
Wild thyme (see page 204) for diverticulitis

Try it in agrimony wine

Put 2 handfuls of flowering agrimony stems and 200 g (8 oz) fresh ginger root or 100 g (4 oz) of the dried root in a large pan with 4.5 litres (1 gallon) water. Bring to the boil and simmer for 25 minutes. Put 1.5 kg (3 lb) white sugar and the zest and juice of 3 oranges and 3 lemons into a bucket, and strain onto it the agrimony and ginger liquid. Stir until the sugar dissolves and when cool add 1 sachet of wine yeast. Cover and leave for three days, then strain into a demijohn, fit an airlock and leave until fermentation ceases. Bottle and leave for at least six months before drinking. Take a wineglassful for an upset stomach.

Agrimony

Forager's checklist

❊ **Perennial herb**

❊ **Widely distributed**

❊ **Tall flower spikes**

❊ **Gentle astringent**

❊ **Fresh or dried herb effective**

❊ **Harvest the whole herb**

❊ **Look for the seed burs on clothes and animals**

❊ **Up to 1 m (3 ft) high**

❊ **Family: Rosaceae**

Agropyron repens

Couch grass

dog grass, twitch grass

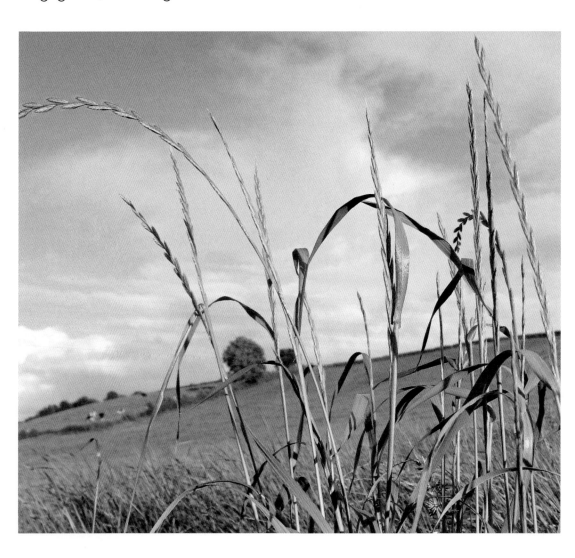

Fact and folklore

Couch grass is detested by gardeners as it is so difficult to eliminate, with the smallest piece of root quickly growing and establishing many new plants. It is also known as dog grass because dogs seek it out to eat when they are unwell; the 17th-century herbalist Nicholas Culpeper said that you can identify this plant by observing which grasses dogs eat. The grass was taken traditionally as a remedy for gall bladder problems and was reputed to prevent stones; it does have some bitter properties that seem to support this use, but it is not commonly used for this by modern herbalists. The roots grow prolifically, and in Italy they are often gathered and eaten for their pleasant sweet flavour.

The plant is rich in chromium, selenium, silicon, phosphorus, magnesium and manganese. Chromium is an important element for the regulation of insulin in the body. Silicon and phosphorus are both essential for bone and connective tissue repair and health. The rhizomes contain mucilage, which has soothing properties and can be used for inflammation and pain in the urinary tract caused by infections and by kidney stones. It is also diuretic and will help to flush out infective bacteria and stones. These properties also make it of value to help ease the symptoms of prostate disease, such as poor urine flow. Its diuretic properties also mean it can assist with the removal of joint-irritating acids that cause the inflammation and pain of gout.

What to look for

It forms large clumps of grass, 60–100 cm (2–3 ft) tall, with shallow, wide-spreading, yellowy-white, rhizomatous roots, with nodules at 5–7.5 cm (2–3 in) intervals from which it sends up new plantlets. The

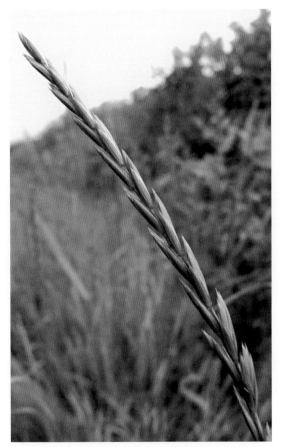

The seedheads of couch grass emerge slightly later than other meadow grasses; it is their distinguishing feature.

Couch grass

leaves are long and thin, and the stems have thickened joints, at regular intervals, that snap cleanly off. The pointed seedheads form in flat rows on either side at the top of the stem and contain many seeds.

Can be mistaken for

Rye grass (*Lolium perenne*) is similar, but the seeds have open-splayed ends rather than pointed tips.

Where to look

Couch grass grows on the edges of arable fields, meadows and on waste ground, and frequently invades the loose fertile soil of flowerbeds and vegetable patches in gardens.

When to look for it

Couch grass grows all year round; it flowers and produces seed in July.

What to harvest

The roots in spring or autumn.

What is it good for?

Gout • Cystitis • Kidney stones • Prostate problems

How to use it

Dig up the roots and make a fresh herb tincture for use alone or in combination with other tinctures. The roots may be dried for use in infusions that are more suited to urinary treatments. Take the warm infusion freely for cystitis and to flush out kidney stones. Combine it with nettles for gout. Use the tincture in combination with other herbs for prostate problems. Cook the fresh roots either by stir frying or simmering in water for ten minutes. They can then be eaten as a vegetable.

Cautions

None.

Combines well with

Wild thyme (see page 204) and yarrow (see page 84) for cystitis
Nettle root (see page 155) for prostate problems
Dandelion leaf (see page 114) for kidney stones

Forager's checklist

❋ Invasive perennial grass
❋ Widely distributed
❋ Tall grass clumps
❋ Use the rhizomes
❋ Harvest in spring or autumn
❋ Urinary demulcent
❋ 60–100 cm (2–3 ft) high and 30 cm (1 ft) wide
❋ Family: Gramineae/Poaceae

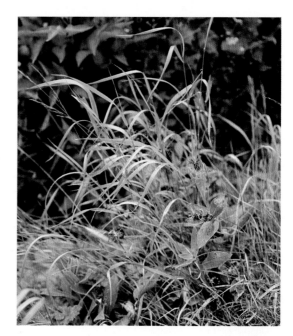

Large clumps of grass that persist well into the autumn when other grasses have died back are often couch grass.

Avena sativa

Oat

wild oat, groats, common oat

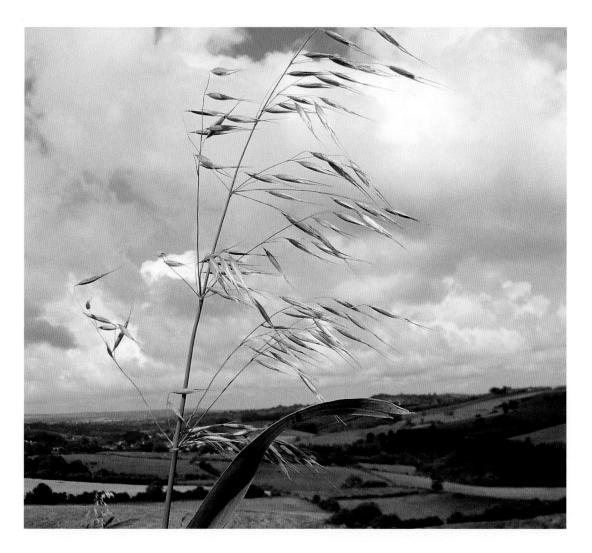

Fact and folklore

Oats have been cultivated for hundreds of years and there are about 25 varieties grown. Cultivated escapees are found growing on the margins and among the main crop of arable fields alongside wild oats. Commercially harvested oats are known as groats, which are prepared for eating by steaming and rolling them. Oats' medicinal virtues are gained by eating them as food. Combine with protein to prolong the energy released. Oats also have emollient properties that are helpful in dry, itchy skin conditions.

Oats are food for the nerves, to be used in any situation when the nervous system is under strain and its resources are being depleted. Oats are a valuable restorative if depression is already an issue, but they are also invaluable during stressful times to support and nourish and prevent nervous collapse. Also take them for convalescence after acute illness or during chronic illness for support, especially diseases of the nerves such as shingles and herpes.

What to look for

A tall plant, 1.2 m (4 ft) high, with grass-like stems and leaves. The seeds hang down from a thin, tough stem emerging from the top of the plant. The true wild oat has a split seed; the bottom half bears an 'awl', which is a long stalk.

Can be mistaken for

The common wild oat (*Avena fatua*) is similar except that both halves of the seed bear an awl. It has the same medicinal properties as *A. sativa*.

Where to look

Oats can be found in field margins of arable crops, hedgerows and meadows.

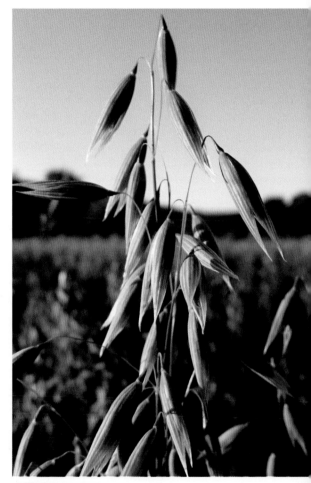

Both cultivated oats (*Avena sativa*) and wild oats (*Avena fatua*) may be used medicinally.

When to look for it
Oats produce seeds in July and August.

What to harvest
The whole plant, when the seed 'pops' and exudes a milky juice when squeezed between the fingers.

What is it good for?
Cold sores • Cramp • Osteoporosis • Restless leg syndrome • Anaemia • High cholesterol • Anxiety and stress • Chickenpox and shingles • Depression • Exhaustion • Insomnia • Neuralgia • Menopause • Premenstrual tension (PMT)

How to use it
The tincture may be made from the oat straw or grass. The easiest method, which preserves the best of the oats' qualities, is to harvest the whole plant and make a fresh herb tincture. Take it for all situations when the nerves are under strain. A handful of porridge oats in an old stocking can be used in the bath for emollient moisturizing effects.

Cautions
Do not take oats if you have coeliac disease or gluten allergy. If treating severe depression, it is advisable to do so with the assistance of a registered medical herbalist and your doctor. Do not cease taking any prescribed medications for depression or anxiety without consultation with your doctor.

Combines well with
St John's wort (see page 137) and wood betony (see page 111) for depression, anxiety, menopausal or premenstrual anxiety, shingles and herpes
Nettle seed (see page 155) for adrenal exhaustion

Forager's checklist
❊ **Annual cereal crop**
❊ **Widely distributed in the wild**
❊ **Tall grass with pendulous seeds**
❊ **Prime nerve restorative**
❊ **Fresh green leaves and stem are best for tincture**
❊ **Harvest the whole plant in summer**
❊ **Cut stems with scissors as they can cut your skin when plucked**
❊ **1–2 m (4 ft) high**
❊ **Family: Gramineae/Poaceae**

Oat

Try it in oat milk
Milk made from oats is a pleasant, nerve-nourishing alternative to cow's milk. Soak 1 part oatmeal in 10 parts water overnight. Put in a food processor or liquidizer and blend for a minute. Strain through a muslin or jelly bag and squeeze out all the liquid. Add water, to taste, to the liquid. If you can obtain whole oats (also called groats), you can sprout them first before making them into milk. They are rich in nutritious enzymes. Soak them overnight in a jar, strain the water off in the morning and leave them in a light place to start growing. This usually takes one to two days. When they have a small shoot emerging, process in a blender as before, ratios being 1 part sprouted oats to 4 parts water. Store the milk in the refrigerator and use within two days.

Euphrasia officinalis
Eyebright
Casse-lunette

Grassland plants

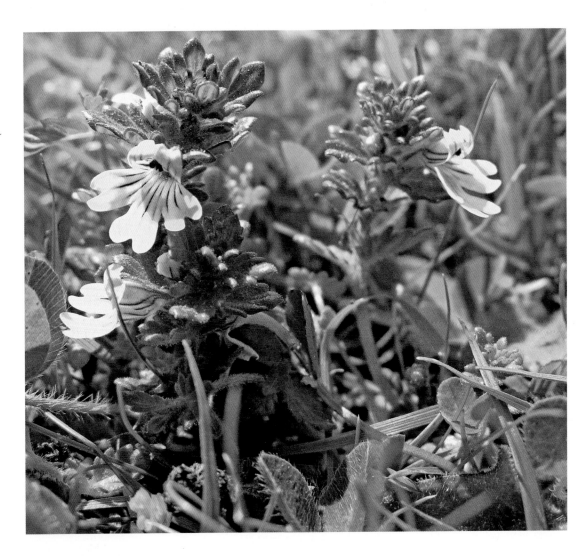

Fact and folklore

It is said that eyebright was named after one of the three muses, Euphrosyne, who represented joy and gladness. The plant has a long tradition for treating poor eyesight, and continues to be used by herbalists for the same thing today. Eyebright is rich in tannins, which help to tighten inflamed mucous membranes, reducing the ability of irritants to aggravate further, and also reducing the amount of mucus produced. The herb is also bitter, and this works via the liver to modify over-active immune responses and to reduce any excess toxins putting a strain on the system. So it is a mucous membrane tonic that can be used to combat the uncomfortable, itchy, watery eyes and nose symptomatic of hayfever and allergies, and also for eye infections.

What to look for

Eyebright is a small annual plant, growing close to the ground, 10–20 cm (4–8 in) high and 15 cm (6 in) wide, with deeply cut leaves. It bears small, unusually shaped flowers, with a three-lobed lower lip and a double-lobed upper lip; the lobes are notched. The flowers are white with dark purple spots and a yellow-splashed centre. The dark spot is a sign of the Doctrine of Signatures and is supposed to resemble the eye.

Can be mistaken for

There are several different species of eyebright growing throughout Europe, but they are all interchangeable medicinally.

Where to look

Eyebright is semi-parasitic on grass, so is only found in dry, grassy areas, especially heathland.

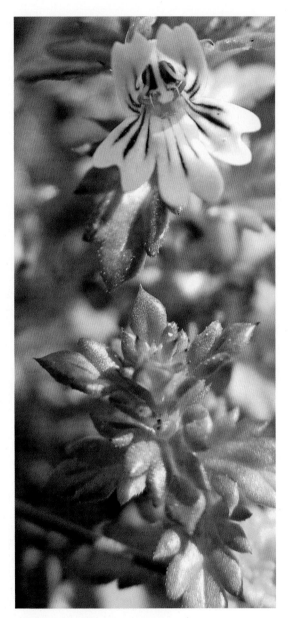

Eyebright will only grow in conjunction with grasses – usually in well-grazed meadows.

When to look for it

Eyebright grows from June through to September. It can be quite difficult to spot until it starts to flower.

What to harvest

The whole flowering plant.

What is it good for?

Conjunctivitis • Catarrh • Hayfever

How to use it

Dry it for use in infusions. Make an infusion and use as an eyewash three times a day for irritated or infected eyes. Keep a small amount in a dropper bottle to carry around and use 4 drops in the affected eye, every two hours if the problem is severe. Discard and replace with a fresh infusion every day. Take the infusion internally for catarrh or hayfever and allergic symptoms of itching throat and itchy, runny nose. The tincture is an effective way to store the herb, which loses some effectiveness on drying. Dilute 2 drops of eyebright tincture in an eyebath of warm water and use to rinse eyes up to six times a day.

Cautions

This is a gentle herb, but do not risk your eyesight. If you are unsure of what you are treating, get a formal diagnosis and professional advice. Corneal abrasions and tears from accidents or objects poked in the eye need consultation with an ophthalmic specialist.

Combines well with

Ground ivy (see page 175), plantain (see page 105) and nettle (see page 155) for hayfever and catarrh
Ground ivy (see page 175), dog rose petals (see page 143) and chamomile (see page 102) as an eyebath

Forager's checklist

❋ **Annual herb**

❋ **Widely distributed**

❋ **Eye-catching flowers**

❋ **Eye tonic**

❋ **Partially parasitic on grass**

❋ **Harvest whole plants**

❋ **10–20 cm (4–8 in) high and 15 cm (6 in) wide**

❋ **Family: Scrophulariaceae**

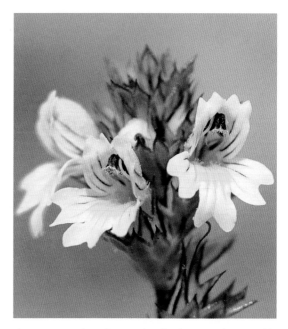

The tiny eye-catching flowers of eyebright are said to resemble the eye, a good example of the Doctrine of Signatures.

Fumaria officinalis

Fumitory

earth smoke

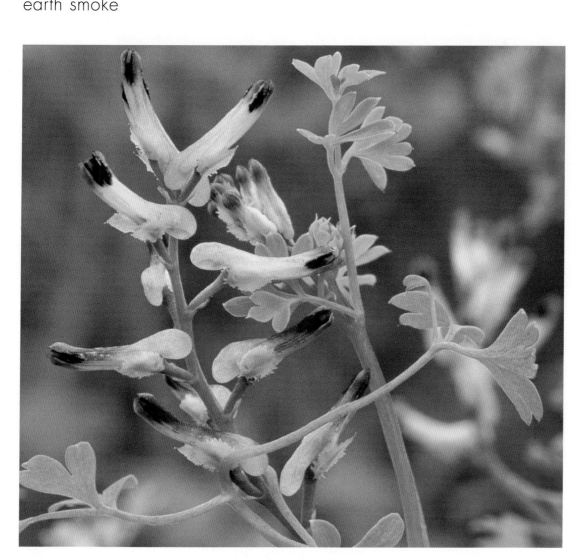

Grassland plants

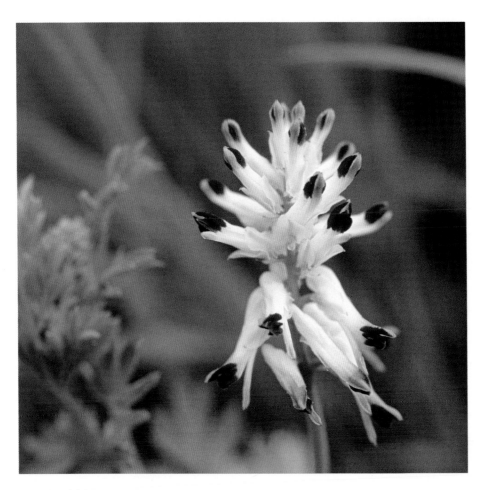

Fumitory scrambles over other grasses and plants around it, with the pretty flowers held high for pollinators.

Fact and folklore

Fumitory is also called earth smoke because of the wispy, smoke-like appearance its foliage has as it grows. Legend says that it formed not from a plant but from vapours rising from the earth. Fumitory was traditionally used for the treatment of liver disorders and skin infections. It is a bitter plant that stimulates the liver to produce more bile. This helps to flush through the bile duct, which may ease the passage of gallstones that are causing symptoms. Its liver-stimulating properties will encourage removal of waste products from the body, making it useful for skin diseases such as eczema and psoriasis. Any plant that stimulates bile production and the liver will also gently stimulate the bowel, making it useful for treating constipation.

What to look for

Fumitory is an annual plant that grows 15–30 cm (6–12 in) high and wide. It has pale green-grey leaves that are deeply cut into three lobes, each with toothed edges. They are borne on weak, straggly stems that scramble up and over other plants. The flowers are thin, tube-like and deep pinky-red with darker lips.

Can be mistaken for

There are many subspecies of fumitory that have the same medicinal qualities. The tube-like flower shape is similar to the flowers of the pea family, like the vetches, but those are pointed at the lower end whereas the flowers of fumitory are rounded.

Where to look

Fumitory is commonly found growing on grassy banks and in ditches, field margins and hedgerows.

When to look for it

It grows from April and flowers from June to September.

What to harvest

The whole flowering plant.

What is it good for?

Acne rosacea • Acne vulgaris • Boils • Psoriasis • Constipation • Gallstones

How to use it

Fumitory makes a good fresh herb tincture because its bitterness may make it unpalatable as an infusion. Take the tincture for gallstones and sluggish liver function. Use it for skin infection or chronic skin disease, such as acne and eczema.

Forager's checklist

* ❋ **Annual weed**
* ❋ **Widely distributed**
* ❋ **Thin, tube-like flowers**
* ❋ **Found on banks and in ditches**
* ❋ **Fresh herb tincture is the best preparation**
* ❋ **Harvest the whole plant when in flower**
* ❋ **Liver tonic**
* ❋ **15–30 cm (6–12 in) high and wide**
* ❋ **Family: Fumariaceae**

Cautions

Be aware of the risk of acute impaction of gallstones. If impaction is suspected, contact your doctor. The risk is theoretically reduced by an increased production of thin bile, as stones will settle to the bottom of the gall bladder and the thinner bile is ejected more easily when required for digestion.

Combines well with

Cramp bark (see page 187) for gallstones
Wild thyme (see page 204) as a skin wash for infections

Try it in fumitory lotion

Use this as a wash, up to three times a day, for weeping skin conditions. Make an infusion of 25 g (1 oz) dried fumitory (50 g (2 oz) fresh herb) to 600 ml (1 pint) boiling water. Leave to infuse for at least 10 minutes. Strain and apply to the affected area with cotton wool. Store in the refrigerator and use within 36 hours.

Matricaria recutita / Chamaemelum nobile

Chamomile

german chamomile, roman chamomile

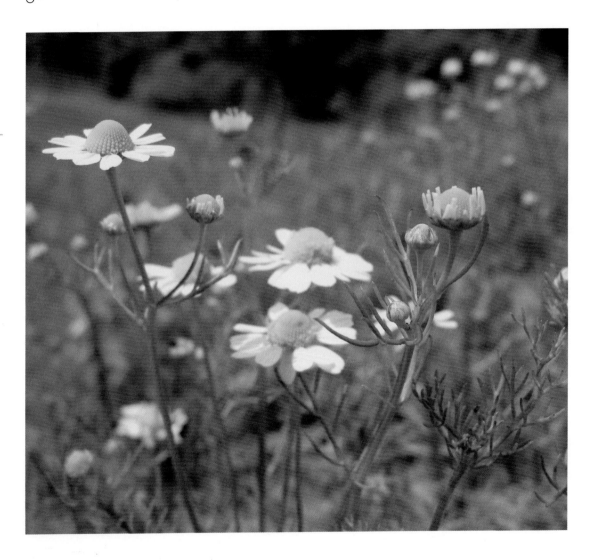

Fact and folklore

There are two types of chamomile used medicinally: the annual German chamomile (*Matricaria recutita*), which has scented flowers, and the perennial Roman chamomile (*Chamaemelum nobile*), which is scented all over. The name comes from the Greeks, who thought it had the scent of apples – hence *khamaimelon*, *khama* meaning 'on the ground' and *melon* meaning 'apple'.

Both plants have gentle sedative and relaxant properties that are used for many conditions, particularly those of the digestive tract. They are gentle enough to be used for babies and children. They are also anti-allergenic and anti-inflammatory and used for irritating skin conditions such as eczema and inflammation of the digestive tract. Roman chamomile is more bitter than German chamomile; it will relax stressed nerves but also stimulate the liver to help eliminate excess stress hormones and improve digestion.

What to look for

Both plants grow 20–30 cm (8–12 in) high and 30 cm (12 in) wide. The leaves of the two plants look similar and are deeply cut, those of Roman chamomile being scented and those of the German chamomile unscented. Roman chamomile emerges from existing stems and German chamomile grows from seed each spring. German chamomile grows taller and more branching, with delicate, hollow flowers at the end of stems that have occasional leaves at their base. Roman chamomile has a creeping habit, the rosettes of leaves remaining low to the ground and the solid flowers, often with double petals, at the end of leafless stems. The flowers of both types of chamomile are small and resemble daisies, with distinctive white petals and a yellow centre.

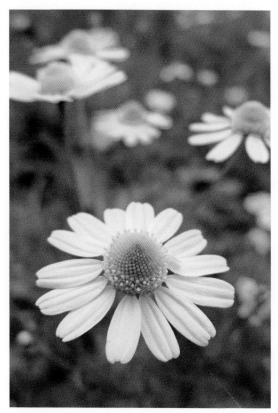

When split carefully in half, the hollow centre of the domed head of German chamomile may be seen.

Can be mistaken for

The scent is a good distinguishing factor. Corn chamomile (*Anthemis arvensis*) has no scent. Stinking chamomile or mayweed (*A. cotula*) is unpleasantly scented. Scentless chamomile or sea mayweed (*Tripleurospermum maritimum*) is found at the seaside.

Where to look

Chamomile grows in well-drained soil on waste ground and around field margins.

When to look for it

It grows from April to October and flowers from June to September.

What to harvest

The flowers.

What is it good for?

Acne rosacea • Acne vulgaris • Bites and stings • Conjunctivitis • Eczema • Cramp • Restless leg syndrome • Earache • Hayfever • Anxiety and stress • Chickenpox and shingles • Headache • Insomnia • Allergies • Fever • Colic • Diarrhoea • Flatulence • Hangover • Heartburn • Indigestion • Irritable bowel syndrome (IBS) • Nausea • Painful periods

How to use it

Collect the flowers of either plant and make a fresh herb tincture for use as a simple or in combination with other herbs. Dry the flowers for use in infusions, eye and skin washes and compresses for its relaxing and anti inflammatory healing properties. The infusion of German chamomile may be added to baths, which is particularly useful for young babies. Roman chamomile is bitter to drink as a tea so is not suitable for children. Make an infused oil of the fresh flowers for topical use on inflamed skin and also to be used as eardrops. Roman chamomile is more commonly used externally. German chamomile is more suited to internal use.

Cautions

Do not take Roman chamomile during pregnancy. Be careful with therapeutic doses of chamomile in combination if warfarin or orthodox anticoagulants are being taken.

Combines well with

Meadowsweet (see page 169) for indigestion and gastritis
Nettle (see page 155) and dandelion (see page 114) for wet eczema
Plantain (see page 105), chickweed (see page 149) and dandelion (see page 114) for dry eczema

Try it in chickweed and chamomile salve

To make 25 g (1 oz) soft set salve, measure out equal amounts of chickweed-and- chamomile-infused oils to 25 ml (1 fl oz). Put this in a pan and add 5 g (1/4 oz) beeswax. Put the pan on a low heat and melt the beeswax. Test the setting consistency by dipping in a cold spoon. Add more beeswax if a harder salve is required. Pour into a jar and label. Use for itching, inflamed skin conditions as required. This will keep for up to a year. Discard if it smells rancid.

Forager's checklist

❋ **German chamomile is an annual**

❋ **Roman chamomile is a perennial**

❋ **German chamomile has scented flowers**

❋ **The whole plant of Roman chamomile is scented**

❋ **Widely distributed**

❋ **Gentle relaxant**

❋ **20–30 cm (8–12 in) high and 30 cm (12 in) wide**

❋ **Family: Compositae**

Plantago lanceolata / P. major

Plantain

ribwort plantain, greater plantain, waybread, snakeweed

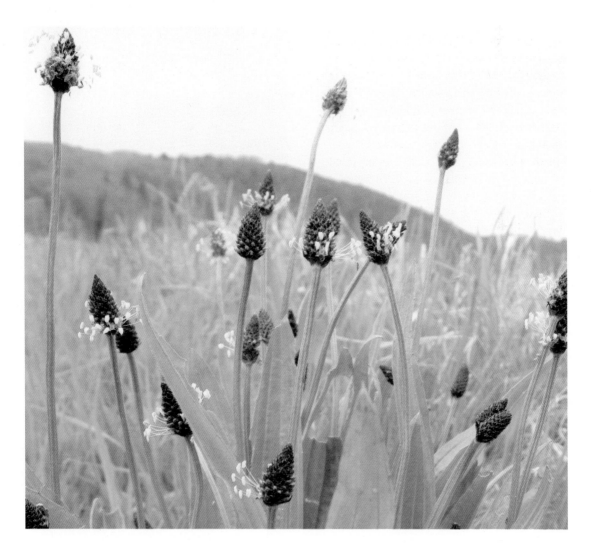

Fact and folklore

The name of ribwort plantain (*P. lanceolata*) alludes to the strong, stringy veins that run through the leaves. Native Americans used the dried root as a remedy to treat snakebite. The leaves are still considered excellent first aid for bites and stings. Externally, the juice is cooling, anti-inflammatory, anti-allergenic and antibacterial. Internally, plantain is a blood cleanser for all toxic, allergic skin conditions. The leaves of greater plantain (*P. major*) are rich in the trace element quercetin, which has been shown to have antihistamine effects in the body and can help to reduce the symptoms of allergies. It is also used for bleeding, irritated conditions of the mucous membranes in the digestive tract, lungs and bladder. Use it for first aid for allergic reactions to bites. It gives almost instant relief from pain and swellings.

What to look for

Greater plantain (*Plantago major*) and ribwort plantain (*P. lanceolata*) are both perennial plants. The leaf shapes of each are different, but unmistakable. They both arise from a basal rosette and grow 15–40 cm (6–16 in) high and 30 cm (12 in) wide. Ribwort plantain has long, lance-shaped leaves, evenly ribbed from base to pointed tip. The flower stalks are angular and the flower is green and cone-shaped with long stamens and purple, pollen-bearing anthers that gradually turn yellow. Greater plantain has large green, round leaves. They resemble the shape of an elephant's ears and have the characteristic plantain vein ribs. The flowering stalk is shorter than that of ribwort and the flower head is longer, with clearer definition of the developing seeds within. The stamen and anthers protrude from the flowering stem in a similar manner to ribwort.

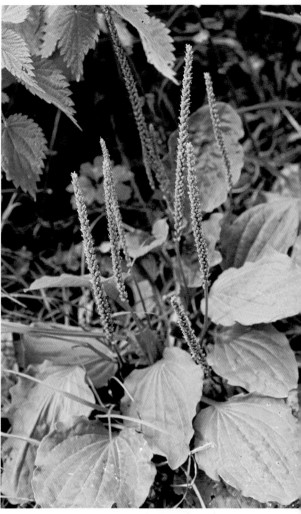

Greater plantain has broad leaves and bears more seeds on its stalks than ribwort plantain (pictured on page 105).

Can be mistaken for

The plants hoary plantain (*Plantago media*) and sea plantain (*P. maritima*) are closely related, and all are interchangeable medicinally.

Where to look

Plantains thrive in most environments and most soils: waste ground, fields, meadows, footpaths and even in our gardens.

When to look for it

The leaves are evergreen but die back to minimal growth during the winter. Plantain flowers from May to September.

What to harvest

The leaves and seeds.

What is it good for?

Bites and stings • Boils • Eczema • Psoriasis • Sunburn • Wounds • Coughs • Earache • Hayfever • Bleeding • Allergies • Constipation • Diarrhoea • Diverticular disease • Hangover • Heartburn • Indigestion • Cystitis • Prostate problems • Incontinence

How to use it

Make an infused oil from the wilted leaves for topical treatment and to use in ointments and salves. Collect the leaves and make a fresh herb tincture to preserve the best of its qualities. It can be dried and used as an infusion, topical wash or poultice. Pick the plant's fresh leaves and pulverize them for use as a poultice, changing it every few hours. Gather and dry the seeds and use 1–2 teaspoons on food as a bulking laxative.

Cautions

Any severe allergic reactions require emergency treatment. Any unusual or prolonged bleeding of bowels or bladder should be immediately investigated by a medical herbalist or doctor to identify the cause.

Plantain

Combines well with

Meadowsweet (see page 169) and chamomile (see page 102) for heartburn
Burdock (see page 125), red clover (see page 117), cleavers (see page 172) and yellow dock (see page 108) for skin disease
Wild thyme (see page 204) and mullein (see page 158) for dry coughs

Try it for first aid sting relief

Rub the fresh leaves hard between your hands until they yield their juice and drop this onto the affected area. Do not rub the bite or sting as this will aggravate the irritation. Repeat as required.

Rumex crispus spp.

Yellow dock

curled dock

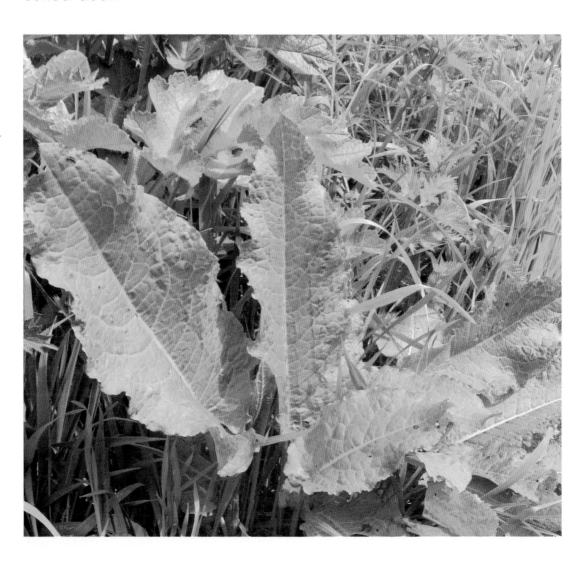

Fact and folklore

One of the most commonly remembered herbal remedies is the dock leaf cure for nettle stings. Yellow dock is so-called because of its yellow roots. According to the Doctrine of Signatures, these indicate bile and their usefulness for treating the liver. Dock is used mainly for treating skin disease by improving the ability of the liver to break down toxins from the system. It is also a gentle laxative and promotes the removal of these waste products from the bowel. It is especially useful in treating elderly people who are constipated and have dry, scaly skin, usually on the legs. It is a specific for itching skin, as this is a sign that the body is trying to eliminate toxins via this route rather than the bowels (and urinary system) and yellow dock will help to remedy this. It also treats anaemia as it improves digestive health and enables the body to better absorb essential minerals like iron.

What to look for

Dock is a perennial plant, 30–60 cm (1–2 ft) high and 30 cm (1 ft) wide, that grows from a thick, yellow taproot. The leaves are narrow and oblong, with wavy edges. They are often tinged with red. Its flowering stem has a few narrow leaves at its base and a branching top with flat, red-hued flowers and seeds.

Can be mistaken for

It is difficult to differentiate from broad-leaved dock (*Rumex obtusifolius*) until it flowers, as the seeds are slightly different in shape. Broad-leaved dock leaves are flatter with less 'curly' edges.

Where to look

Yellow dock grows in rough and waste ground. It is rare in Scotland, but is easily cultivated.

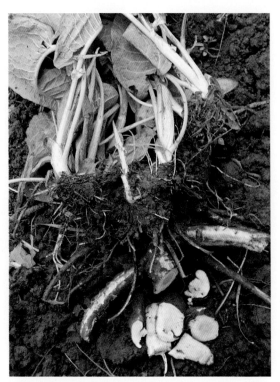

The colour of yellow dock root is a good identifying feature; the yellow also indicates bile and its use for treating the liver.

Yellow dock

When to look for it

The yellow dock produces a basal rosette of leaves in April. It bears flowers in July.

What to harvest

The root in the autumn or early spring.

What is it good for?

Acne vulgaris • Eczema • Psoriasis • Anaemia • Constipation • Diverticular disease

How to use it

Dig up the root in the spring or autumn and make a fresh root tincture. Start taking small doses at first – 1 ml (see page 35) once a day, gradually increasing to three times a day if required. Yellow dock combines well with other herbs for the treatment of skin disease. It can be dried and used as a decoction, but the taste is often found to be unpalatable, bitter and earthy.

Cautions

Big doses may cause diarrhoea. When treating skin disease, always start with small doses to avoid an exacerbation as the body is cleansing itself.

Combines well with

Chickweed (see page 149) and cleavers (see page 172) for dry, itching skin problems
Red clover (see page 117) and dandelion (see page 114) for acne
Yarrow (see page 84) and horse chestnut (see page 38) for varicose eczema seen in old age

Try it in dock leaf nettle cure

It might be that this remedy came from the traditional use of the root in skin disease. It is a good distraction for nettle-stung children to look for dock leaves to apply. Plantain is also effective and yields lots of juice. There is a rhyme to be said when applying a dock to nettle stings:
Nettle in, Dock:
Dock in, Nettle out,
Dock rub Nettle out.

Forager's checklist

* **Self-seeding biennial**
* **Long, wavy-edged leaves**
* **Liver stimulant**
* **Use the yellow root**
* **Harvest in the autumn or early spring**
* **30–60 cm (1–2 ft) high and 30 cm (1 ft) wide**
* **Family: Polygonaceae**

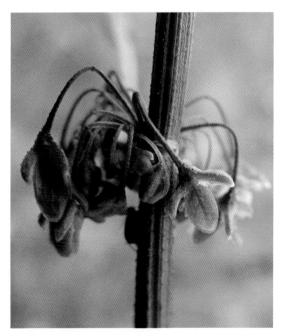

The flowers of yellow dock have rounded edges whereas those of the broad dock have spiked margins.

Stachys betonica

Wood betony

betony

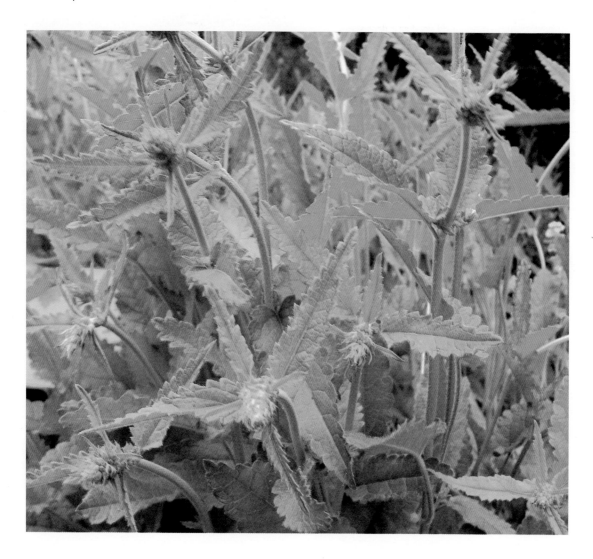

Fact and folklore

Betony has long been held in high esteem as a healer of many ailments. Throughout the history of Europe, from Roman until modern times, there are many sayings and superstitions around its efficacy as a healer. A Roman treatise written by the physician of Emperor Augustus lists it as a cure for 47 diseases. An Italian saying states 'sell your coat and buy betony'.

Wood betony is a gentle nerve relaxant and bitter herb. It is used for headaches, particularly those arising from poor digestion or hangover (liverish) or for those caused by high blood pressure or anxiety and stress, including migraine. It is considered by many herbalists to be a specific for chronic headaches often encountered after head injuries and post concussion. Use it to help the body adapt when stopping regular painkillers for headaches, to support the liver and nerves. It is of value for nervous digestive symptoms such as gastritis and irritable bowel syndrome and is also beneficial for acne rosacea.

What to look for

Wood betony is a perennial plant that grows every spring from a fibrous root system, to 30 cm (1 ft) high. It has many short-stalked, round, toothed leaves at its base and a square stem with occasional unstalked leaves. The flowers grow directly from the stem, mainly at the top in a dense flowerhead. They are pinkish-purple and trumpet-shaped, with a flat upper lip and three-lobed lower lip, arising from a green, spiked calyx.

Can be mistaken for

Marsh woundwort (*Stachys palustris*) has widely spaced, pale pink flowers. Hedge woundwort (*S. sylvatica*) also has widely spaced flowers, more pink than purple, with white markings in the centre. Leaves of both species are oval and pointed. They were both used traditionally as wound herbs.

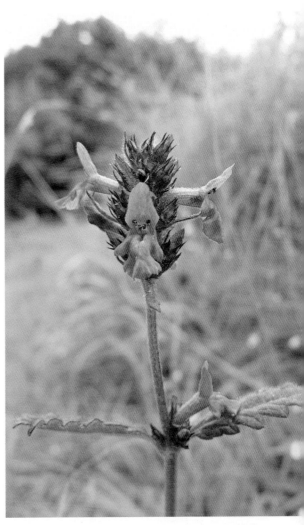

The delicate purple flowers of wood betony are similar to that of woundwort plants, but the leaves are markedly different.

Where to look

Wood betony mainly grows in meadows in partially shaded ground on the edge of woodland or in hedge banks. It may also be found in open grassland.

When to look for it

The plant grows from April to October and flowers from July to September.

What to harvest

The whole flowering plant.

What is it good for?

Acne rosacea • Anxiety and stress • Depression • Headache • Migraine • Irritable bowel syndrome (IBS)

How to use it

Gather the herb just as it is about to flower and dry it for use as an infusion to drink regularly for recurrent headaches or after a meal. Make the fresh herb tincture to include in tincture mixes or to take as a one-off dose at the first sign of a headache. Use the tincture before meals for nervous digestive disorders.

Cautions

If treating high blood pressure, it is advisable to do so with the assistance of a registered medical herbalist and your doctor. Do not stop taking prescribed medications without the assistance of your doctor and a medical herbalist.

Combines well with

Valerian (see page 79) for migraine
Hawthorn (see page 166), lime (see page 56) and mistletoe (see page 59) for headaches associated with high blood pressure

Try it in betony headache blend

Take this infusion for chronic headaches, or make it as a mix of tinctures to take at the first sign of migraine, stress headache or hangover. Blend the following dried herbs or tinctures in equal amounts: wood betony, mint, valerian root, vervain, cramp bark (add 2 ml cramp bark tincture to infusions or decoct it separately. See page 35). Doses are:
Infusion: 25 g (1 oz) to 600 ml (1 pint) water – drink 1 cupful, approximately 200 ml (7 fl oz), three times a day.
Tincture: take 5 ml (1 teaspoon) three times a day for chronic headaches. Take 15 ml ($^1/_2$ fl oz) for acute onset of headache and repeat the dose if necessary an hour later.

Wood betony

Forager's checklist

* **Perennial herb**
* **Widely distributed**
* **Looks similar to hedge and marsh woundwort**
* **Use dried herb**
* **Harvest the whole flowering plant**
* **Tall flower stalks**
* **Digestive nerve tonic**
* **30 cm (1 ft) high**
* **Family: Labiatae**

Taraxacum officinale

Dandelion

lion's tooth, wet the bed, pis en lit

Grassland plants

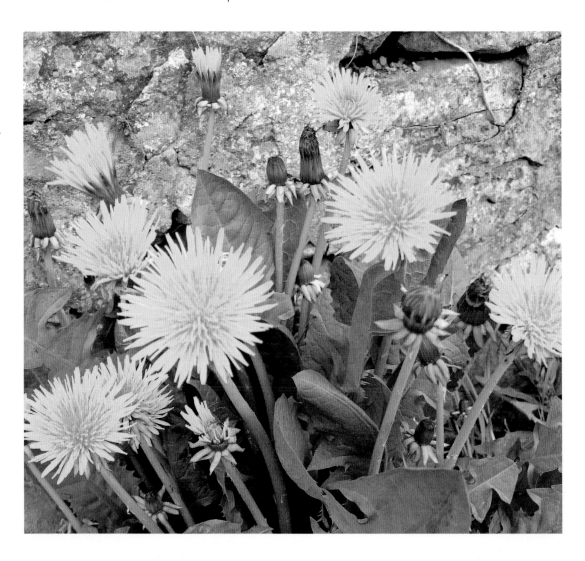

Fact and folklore

The name dandelion comes from the French *dent de lion*, meaning 'lion's tooth', alluding to the shape of the leaves. The strong leaves are high in potassium and have potent diuretic properties that make it a wonderful treatment if you suffer from water retention, high blood pressure or swollen ankles. The bitter root stimulates the liver and the release of enzymes throughout the digestive tract. The dandelion's flower stem exudes a milky-white latex sap that can be applied directly to warts and verrucas to inhibit viral replication. If you suffer from skin problems such as eczema, psoriasis and acne, it can help to flush toxins from the body. Dandelion also has the ability to aid removal of uric acid from the body, making it good for treating gout and joint disease.

What to look for

Dandelion arises from a deep taproot, the smallest part of which, if left in the ground, can grow to form a new plant. It grows to 5–40 cm (2–16 in) high and 30 cm (12 in) wide. Its leaves are deeply saw-toothed, forming a single rosette at the base from which yellow flowers arise, singly, on top of a long, hollow stem that exudes a milky-white sap when broken. The flowers ripen into the 'dandelion clock' – a fluffy ball of wind-borne, umbrella-shaped, feathery filaments, each bearing a seed.

Can be mistaken for

Cat's ear (*Hypochaeris radicata*) is known as false dandelion. It has similar flowers, but the stem is solid and branching and the leaves hairier and deeply lobed.

Where to look

Dandelions thrive in most grassy places: meadows,

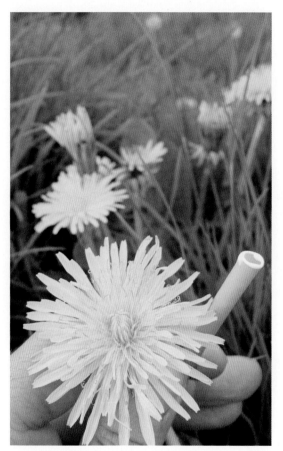

The white sap from the broken flower stems of the dandelion is a specific treatment for warts and verrucas.

cultivated lawns, waste ground and grass verges. This ubiquitous plant is found all over Europe, especially in temperate regions.

When to look for it

You are likely to find dandelions growing all year round. It flowers from March to November but it may continue to flower in a mild winter.

Dandelion

What to harvest

The leaves, roots and sap. The root is best harvested in early spring or autumn when the plant is dormant and before the active growth and flowering depletes its constituents.

What is it good for?

Acne rosacea • Acne vulgaris • Eczema • Psoriasis • Warts and verrucas • Arthritis • Gout • Atherosclerosis • High cholesterol • High blood pressure • Depression • Bloating • Constipation • Flatulence • Gallstones • Indigestion • Irritable bowel syndrome (IBS) • Nausea • Worms • Cystitis • Kidney stones • Menopause • Premenstrual tension (PMT)

How to use it

As soon as the dandelion appears in spring, make the leaves into an infusion or tincture or add them to salads for a spring-clean for the body. The fresh roots can be chopped and made into a tincture or dried for use as a decoction as needed. Apply the sap topically to warts and verrucas on a daily basis (see page 218).

Cautions

Do not use in combination with orthodox diuretics. If treating high blood pressure, it is advisable to do so with the assistance of a medical herbalist and your doctor.

Combines well with

Burdock (see page 125), red clover (see page 117), cleavers (see page 172) and yellow dock (see page 108) for skin disease
Nettle (see page 155) for arthritis and gout

Forager's checklist

* **Frequent lawn plant**
* **Fresh leaves are most potent**
* **Harvest the root in autumn or early spring**
* **Wear gloves while harvesting to avoid the sap staining your skin**
* **Persistent perennial weed**
* **Widely distributed**
* **Saw-toothed leaves**
* **Excellent detoxifier**
* **5–40 cm (2–16 in) high and 30 cm (12 in) wide**
* **Family: Compositae**

Try it in dandelion coffee

This can be used as a coffee substitute. It has a bitter flavour and retains its bitter medicinal properties. Take some fresh roots, chop them and roast at a low temperature for a few hours in the oven until they are brown. Grind as required and use as for ground coffee – 1 teaspoon per mug of boiling water in a cafetière. Do not sweeten, as this reduces the bitter action. The liver needs support in today's modern lifestyle – stress, poor diet and environmental toxins all increase its burden. Dandelion is a useful remedy for daily living.

Trifolium pratense

Red clover

purple clover

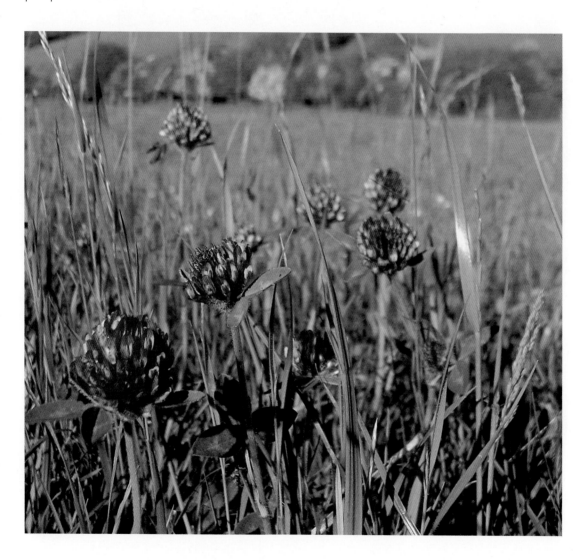

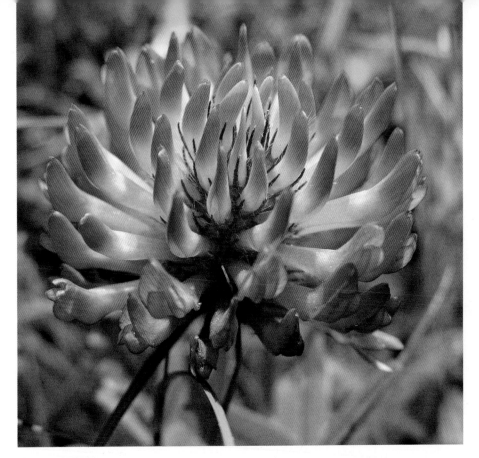

Red clover flowers impart a delicate pink to its wine. They are sweet to eat while walking in the fields.

Fact and folklore

The blossoms harbour a sweet nectar, which you can suck out and savour on your tongue. Red clover has been used in wine-making as well as medicine. It contains plant compounds, isoflavones, that have a similar chemical structure to our own oestrogens, and can play an important role in hormone control. If there is excess oestrogen in the body, red clover inhibits the action of our oestrogen. If there is little or no oestrogen in the body, as in menopause, then red clover provides some oestrogen effect. This is especially useful for skin problems occurring during menopause, such as acne rosacea, and for acne in hormonal teenagers. The skin-cleansing properties of clover are also useful in eczema and psoriasis. Traditionally, it was used as a blood and skin cleanser, and for treating breast cancer, a use which has stimulated scientific interest because of its hormone-modulating effects.

What to look for

Red clover is a short-lived perennial plant, 5–40 cm (2–16 in) high and 30 cm (12 in) wide, that has long, branching stems bearing the typical three-lobed clover leaves, often with white blotches. The oval flowers consist of a multitude of small, trumpet-shaped florets and are deep pink, 2–3 cm (about 1 in) across.

Can be mistaken for
Zigzag clover (*Trifolium medium*) is interchangeable with red clover medicinally.

Where to look
Red clover grows prolifically in pasture and meadows.

When to look for it
You can find red clover from May to October. It flowers in June and July and, if cut, often again in late August or early September.

What to harvest
The flowers.

What is it good for?
Acne rosacea • Acne vulgaris • Eczema • Psoriasis • Enlarged glands • Menopause

How to use it
Harvest the flowers when they are fully open and retaining all of their colour. They are delicious eaten fresh as an ingredient in salads, and may also be dried to be drunk as infusions. The fresh flower tincture is useful in skin disease for combining with root tinctures.

Cautions
Ensure that you dry the flowers rapidly and well – do not allow them to develop any mould as they can ferment and produce anti blood-clotting properties.

Forager's checklist
* **Perennial meadow herb**
* **Widely distributed**
* **Dry the flowers thoroughly**
* **Harvest the flowers in June or July**
* **Common in hay meadows**
* **Three-leaved clover**
* **Gentle skin cleanser**
* **5–40 cm (2–16 in) high and 30 cm (12 in) wide**
* **Family: Papilionaceae**

Red clover

Combines well with
Meadowsweet (see page 169), chamomile (see page 102) and dandelion (see page 114) for acne rosacea
Burdock (see page 125), cleavers (see page 172) and yellow dock (see page 108) for acne vulgaris
Chamomile (see page 102), dandelion (see page 114) and chickweed (see page 149) for eczema

Try it in red clover wine
Gather 4.5 litres (1 gallon) of red clover blossoms. Boil together 1.5 kg (3 lb) sugar and 4.5 litres (1 gallon) water and allow to cool. Pour over the red clover blossoms in a sterile brewing bucket. Add the juice and rind of 3 lemons and 2 oranges. Add 1 sachet of all-purpose wine yeast. Cover and leave in a warm place for five days. Strain into a sterile demijohn and fit an airlock. Leave until fermentation has finished and the wine has cleared. Bottle and leave to mature for at least six months. Take a small glassful every day.

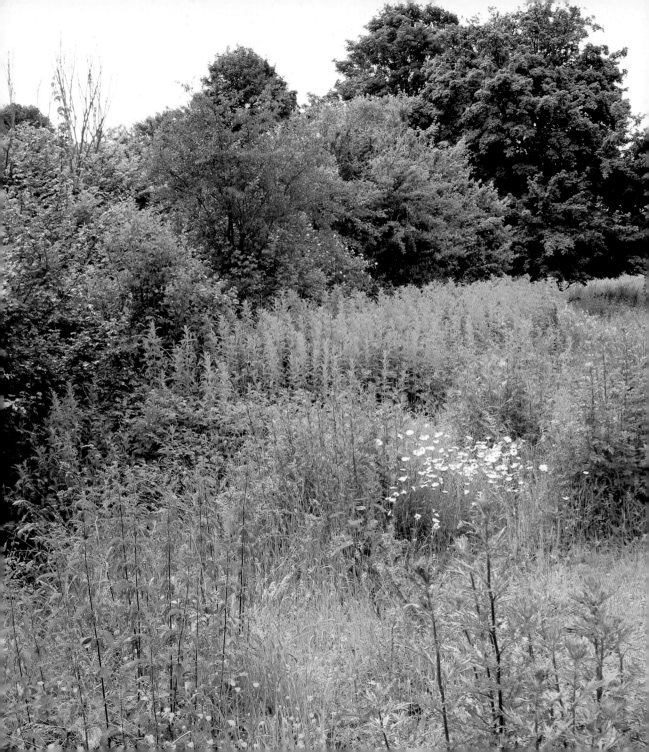

WASTE GROUND PLANTS

Waste ground is surprisingly rich in plant life, and in spring and summer it is transformed into a secret place of abundant growth. Plants that have disappeared from their usual habitats because of chemical use and intensive farming methods colonize such areas and flourish undisturbed. This often over-looked environment can be a solace for an array of beautiful plants and herbs, giving purpose to the space and creating a haven for wildlife.

Armoracia rusticana

Horseradish

moutarde des allemands

Waste ground plants

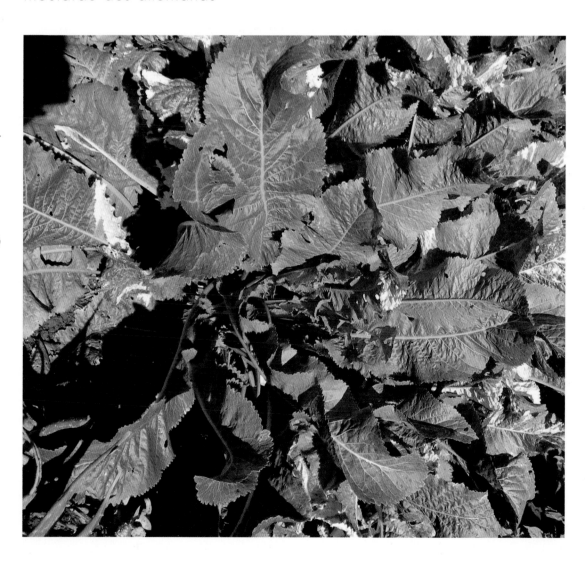

Fact and folklore

The name horseradish distinguishes this plant as a coarse wild radish rather than the cultivated, edible, garden vegetable. In the Middle Ages, the root and leaves were used mainly as a medicine, and its use as a condiment originated in Germany. It is a stimulating and heating herb that is especially useful for cold, damp conditions, promoting blood flow. When you eat a large quantity of horseradish sauce, the pungent, burning smell travels right up your nose, indicating its usefulness in congested sinuses, acute or chronic. The volatile oil is also antiseptic. It is rich in vitamins A and C, potassium, phosphorus and chromium. Used topically, it irritates the tissues so that blood flow is stimulated; this flushes out toxins and provides nutrients to the tissues.

What to look for

Horseradish grows 30–40 cm (12–16 in) high and 60 cm (24 in) wide. It is a perennial plant that has a spreading system of thick roots. It has large, dark green leaves with a distinct crinkly surface that emit the typical pungent horseradish smell when crushed. Many small, four-petalled, white flowers grow on branches at the top of a long stem with narrow leaves.

Can be mistaken for

The leaves of broad-leaved dock (*Rumex obtusifolius*) are smaller and smoother, and do not have the pungent scent.

Where to look

Horseradish grows wild on waste ground and verges.

When to look for it

The plant grows from April to November. When you are out harvesting, replant some of the root crown to produce growth in the following year.

What to harvest

The root in autumn.

What is it good for?

Arthritis • Backache • Cramp • Sprains and strains • Bronchitis • Catarrh • Coughs • Sinusitis • Chilblains • Flatulence • Indigestion

How to use it

Use the root to make horseradish composition (see page 124), or make horseradish sauce and eat it with meals. Make horseradish syrup by covering a piece of fresh grated root with sugar and leaving it for 24 hours; strain off the resulting liquid and keep in the refrigerator. Take 1–2 teaspoons for damp, phlegmy coughs. It will keep for three months. Store the roots in dry sand to keep them fresh over the winter months. Make a poultice with fresh grated root for stiff arthritic joints and chilblains but remove after ten minutes or as soon as it starts to burn (see 'Cautions' below). Make an infused oil and massage it into stiff joints and chilblains, or use it in ointments and liniments.

Cautions

Horseradish should not be taken in cases of gastritis or ulceration of the stomach or intestines. It causes vomiting if taken in excess, and can cause blistering of the skin. Avoid if you suffer from hypothyroidism or if taking thyroxine.

Combines well with

Elecampane (see page 140) as a syrup for bronchitis and catarrh

Horseradish

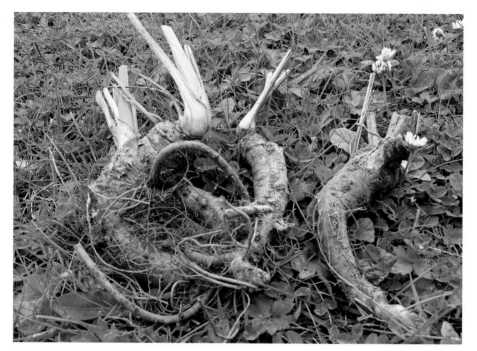

Horseradish roots may be cultivated as an annual vegetable and stored for use during the winter.

Try it in horseradish composition

Peel and thinly slice 25 g (1 oz) fresh horseradish root and place in a wide-necked jar (with a lid), along with $^{1}/_{4}$ teaspoon grated nutmeg and the peel of an organic or wax-free orange. Pour over 100 ml ($3^{1}/_{2}$ fl oz) vodka and close the lid tightly. Shake well. Leave for two weeks, shaking intermittently. Strain, bottle and label. Adults should take 1–2 teaspoons, before meals, for feeble or poor digestion. This will keep like a tincture, for up to three years.

Forager's checklist

* Perennial culinary herb
* Widely distributed
* Large, crinkly leaves
* Pungent smell when crushed
* Root is used
* Digestive stimulant
* 30–40 cm (12–16 in) high and 60 cm (24 in) wide
* Family: Cruciferae

Arctium lappa

Burdock

beggar's buttons

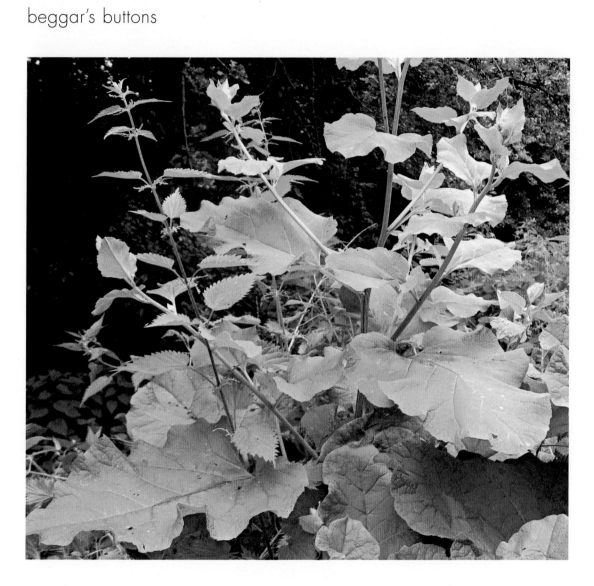

Waste ground plants

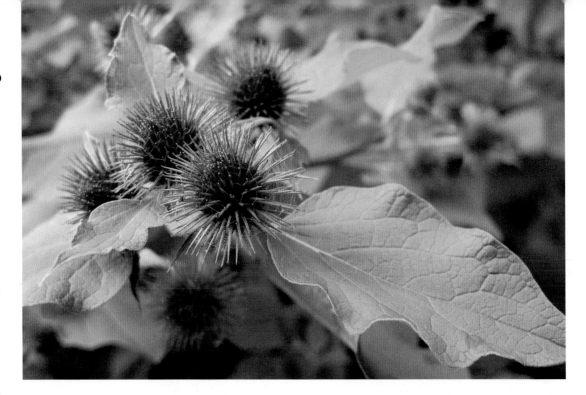

Fact and folklore

The name burdock comes from its prickly seed cases, or burs, and its large leaves, like those of dock. The leaves grow in the first year and it flowers and produces seed in the second. The first-year stems and roots may be cooked and eaten as a vegetable and have a pleasant flavour. The whole plant was once used medicinally but now mainly the root is used. It is diuretic and bitter and so cleansing on the whole system, increasing elimination of toxins that have accumulated through sluggish metabolism and poor diet. Use its cleansing actions for skin and joint disease and constipation. It also soothes the digestive tract and restricts the absorption of further toxins. It is also rich in chromium and other minerals and may be of use in insulin-resistant conditions and cases of high blood-sugar levels.

Beware the ripe, clingy burs of burdock as they contain tiny hairs that are very irritating to the skin.

What to look for

Burdock is a biennial plant that grows 60–200 cm (2–8 ft) high and 60 cm (2 ft) wide. It arises from a deep, thick taproot and in its first year produces a rosette of large, wavy-edged leaves that are green on top, pale underneath and covered with a fine down. In the second year, a tall flower spike emerges, bearing large, green flowers with a scaled calyx and many lilac florets in the centre. These then form the seedheads and the calyx dries into a sticky bur that clings to passing objects, enabling them to be dispersed.

Can be mistaken for

The leaves of broad-leaved dock (*Rumex obtusifolius*)

are oval and without the wavy-edged margins and pale undersides seen on burdock.

Where to look
Burdock thrives in damp ground by rivers and streams and on waste ground.

When to look for it
It grows from March to October.

What to harvest
The root in the first year.

What is it good for?
Acne vulgaris • Boils • Eczema • Psoriasis • Arthritis • Gout • Constipation

How to use it
Make a fresh root tincture. For eczema, psoriasis and acne, begin by taking small 1 ml doses (see page 35) and increase the amount and frequency slowly. This will avoid rapid elimination of toxins that can make skin conditions worse. The root may also be dried. Take a decoction for arthritic conditions, gout and constipation to increase the diuretic effect and flush out waste products. Take either the decoction or tincture regularly for insulin resistance and high blood-sugar levels.

Cautions
Take only small doses to begin with, to avoid aggravating skin problems such as eczema.

Combines well with
Yellow dock (see page 108) and dandelion (see page 114) for constipation

Red clover (see page 117), cleavers (see page 172) and dandelion (see page 114) for acne
Nettle (see page 155) for insulin resistance

Try it in dandelion and burdock beer
Put 500 g (1 lb) fresh young nettles, 100 g (4 oz) fresh dandelion leaves, 100 g (4 oz) fresh burdock root (50 g/2 oz dried), peeled and sliced, the rind of 2 lemons and 25 g (1 oz) fresh or 12.5 g ($^1/_2$ oz) dried ginger root into a pan with 4.5 litres (1 gallon) water. Bring to the boil and simmer for 30 minutes. Put the juice of 2 lemons, 500 g (1 lb) brown sugar and 25 g (1 oz) cream of tartar into a bucket and strain in the boiled nettle mixture, pressing out all the liquid. Stir until the sugar is dissolved. Allow to cool and add 1 sachet brewing yeast. Cover and allow to ferment in a warm place for three to four days. Then bottle, adding 1 teaspoon sugar to each bottle. Leave the bottles for at least a week until the beer has cleared.

Burdock

Forager's checklist
* **Biennial herb**
* **Widely distributed**
* **Large, clingy burs**
* **Blood cleanser**
* **Long taproot**
* **Harvest root in the first year**
* **60–200 cm (2–8 ft) high and 60 cm (2 ft) wide**
* **Family: Compositae**

Artemisia vulgaris

Mugwort

felon herb

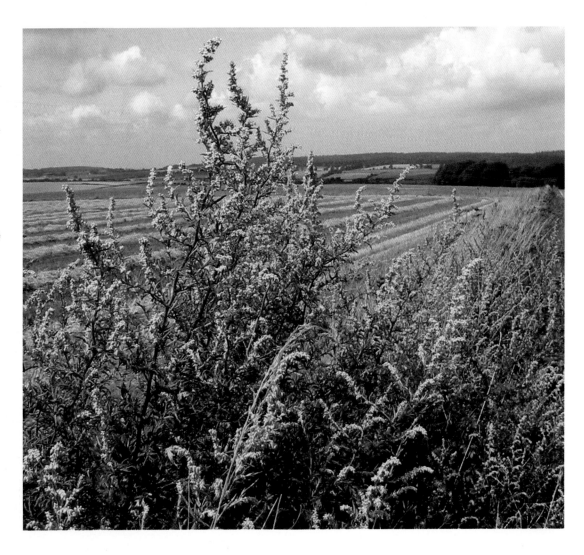

Fact and folklore

Artemisia is named after the Greek moon goddess, Artemis. The herbalist Culpeper said it was a plant of Venus, continuing its association with strong, female energy. Because mugwort was said to protect the traveller from evil doings, wild beasts and becoming footsore, people walking long distances would put a leaf inside their shoe. It is used in Chinese medicine as moxa, where the leaf is dried and then finely shredded until it produces a fine, fluffy powder. This is formed into cones or tightly bound sticks. It is burned on or near the skin to stimulate heat and circulation and increase Qi or energy in stagnant conditions.

Mugwort is a bitter herb used to stimulate appetite and digestion for anorexia, poor appetite or for indigestion and digestive fullness after eating. It also has antispasmodic properties and can be taken to ease period pains. It can help to bring on a menstrual period that is slow to start, especially one that is painful before the bleeding commences due to sluggish pelvic blood flow. It also has mildly relaxing properties that may help with associated anxiety and tension, and it has a reputation for inducing dreams, when taken before bed. A hot infusion will also induce sweating, making it useful for fevers and infections, especially of the female reproductive system. It is also considered to have antiparasitic properties, particularly against intestinal worms.

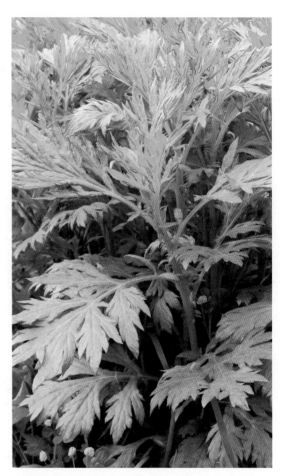

Mugwort has many medicinal family members including wormwood, southernwood and sweet Annie.

What to look for

Mugwort is a tall, shrubby perennial that has long, angled, branching stems from its base, 60–120 cm (2–4 ft) high and 30 cm (1 ft) wide. The stems are often tinged with red. The deeply cut, toothed leaves are dark green on the upperside and almost white with a fine, felt-like coating underneath. The many flowers are yellowy-brown, small and oval, and borne on tall spikes. The whole plant has a pungent scent.

Can be mistaken for

The highly aromatic wormwood (*Artemisia absinthium*) has silvery-green foliage and yellow flowers, and is intensely bitter and fragrant.

Mugwort

Where to look

Mugwort is commonly found growing on grass verges, footpaths and on waste ground.

When to look for it

It grows from April to October and flowers from July to September.

What to harvest

The whole flowering plant.

What is it good for?

Bruises • Insomnia • Fever • Indigestion • Worms • Painful periods

How to use it

Gather and dry the plant when it is just about to flower for use in an infusion. Use a smaller than standard dose for infusion: 12.5 g (1/2 oz) of dried herb to 600 ml (1 pint) water. Take it hot for sluggish periods and congestive period pain. Make the fresh herb tincture for use in small doses in combination with other herbs. The dose for mugwort tincture is less than standard tincture doses: 1 ml (see page 35) up to three times a day should suffice.

Cautions

Do not use mugwort during pregnancy.

Combines well with

Yarrow (see page 84) for periods that are delayed, slow or painful

Forager's checklist

※ **Perennial wayside herb**

※ **Widely distributed**

※ **Bitter tonic**

※ **Use the dried herb**

※ **Harvest when in flower**

※ **60–120 cm (2–4 ft) high and 30 cm (1 ft) wide**

※ **Family: Compositae**

Try it in home-made moxa sticks

Gather and dry some mugwort. Strip the leaves from the stems and crumble them as finely as possible. Use a pestle and mortar to grind them into a fine, fluffy powder. Pack the resulting powder into a large cigarette paper and roll it up as tightly as possible. Use this for old bruises, strains and fibrous muscular injuries that persist long after the initial injury. Light the end and blow out the flame, leaving burning embers. Hold this above the affected area and move it in small circles, allowing the heat to penetrate for five minutes, twice a day. It will smoke so do this treatment outside or in a well-ventilated room. The area will feel unusually warm after this treatment; it opens up the flow of energy and facilitates healing.

Capsella bursa-pastoris

Shepherd's purse

witches' pouches, mother's heart

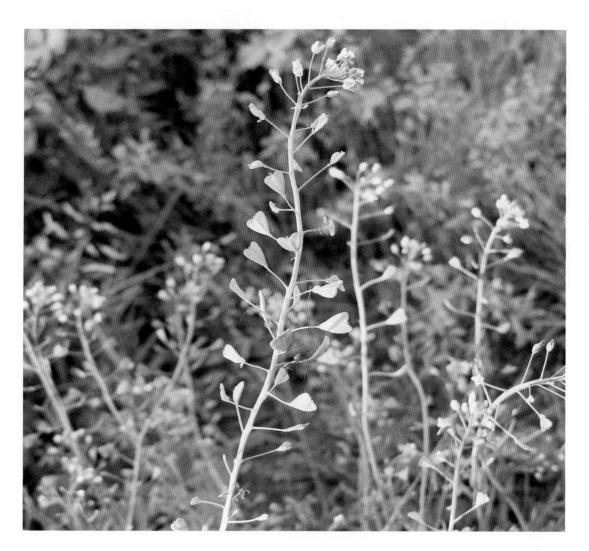

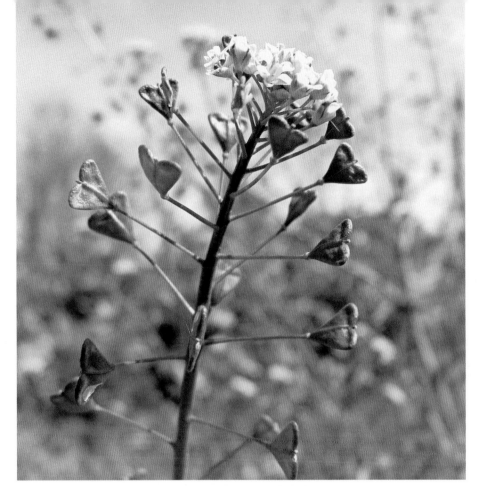

The delicate heart-shaped seedpods of shepherd's purse are a good identifying feature and give it its name.

Fact and folklore

This plant is called shepherd's purse because of its resemblance to old-fashioned leather money pouches. Its Latin name also relates to this, and to the fact that it commonly grows in pastures. It has been used for its tannins and astringent properties for hundreds of years. It was an important herb in the First World War, being used to reduce and stop bleeding from wounds. Modern herbalists still consider it to be an important ally in the treatment of bleeding from anywhere in the body, including the gums, bowels and bladder, and it is most commonly used for excessive menstrual bleeding. It is also useful in the treatment of diarrhoea that persists after a bout of food poisoning when the intestine and bowel walls are inflamed. When persistent coughing or vomiting has caused a small tear in the back of the throat or larynx and streaks of fresh blood are present in the vomit or saliva, shepherd's purse is useful as a gargle to close the exposed blood vessels.

What to look for

Shepherd's purse may be an annual or biennial plant depending on when it sets its seed. It grows 20–40 cm (8–16 in) high. It has deeply cut leaves, 5 cm (2 in) long, that grow mainly in a basal rosette; from this rises the flower stem, which is round and branching at the top. The whole plant bears sparse hairs. The four-petalled flowers are small and dirty white, and these develop into the distinctive, small, heart-shaped seedpods that are notched down the middle – inside, the seeds are attached along this notch.

Can be mistaken for

The basal leaves and stem bear a resemblance to those of hairy bittercress (*Cardamine hirsuta*), but that plant is generally much smaller and the seedpods are elongated rather than heart-shaped.

Where to look

Shepherd's purse grows in many different soils – even the driest crevice with little or poor soil, although it may not grow to a great height – in gardens, meadows and pasture, on waste ground and along footpaths.

When to look for it

You are likely to find shepherd's purse growing all year round. It flowers from March to November.

What to harvest

The whole flowering plant.

What is it good for?

Gums and teeth • Sore throat • Anaemia • Bleeding • Haemorrhoids (piles) • Nosebleed • Diarrhoea • Cystitis • Incontinence • Heavy periods

Forager's checklist

* ❄ **Annual weed**
* ❄ **Widely distributed**
* ❄ **Use the whole plant**
* ❄ **Harvest when in flower**
* ❄ **Heart-shaped seedpods**
* ❄ **Antihaemorrhagic**
* ❄ **20–40 cm (8–16 in) high**
* ❄ **Family: Cruciferae**

How to use it

Gather the herb and use it fresh, or dry it for use in infusions to drink for diarrhoea, heavy periods and blood in the urine. Allow the infusions to cool and use as a mouthwash for gum disease, a gargle for sore throats, a compress or enema for bleeding piles and as a douche for non-infective vaginal discharge. Alternatively, make a fresh herb tincture for combining with other herbs. Soak a piece of gauze in the fresh juice, infusion or diluted tincture and insert into the nostril to stop a nosebleed.

Cautions

Any persistent or unexplained bleeding should be investigated by your doctor or a medical herbalist.

Combines well with

Silverweed (see page 70) for heavy periods
Wood avens (see page 44) as a mouthwash for bleeding gums

Shepherd's purse

Chelidonium majus

Celandine

greater celandine

Fact and folklore

Celandine starts to flower at the time the swallows arrive and stops when they leave, which may be why the Greeks named it *chelidon*, meaning 'swallow'. Pliny writes that the swallows discovered its properties and used it for treating the eyes of their chicks.

Traditionally, the sap was mixed in milk and used as a wash to remove opaque films over the cornea of the eye. The sap is bright orange and will leave a brown stain on the skin. The Doctrine of Signatures says that this colour indicates the bile and the liver. The alkaloids in the sap inhibit cell replication, making it effective for treating warts, verrucas and fungal infections such as ringworm. It has also been investigated for use in the treatment of some cancers.

It is irritant and caustic, so avoid getting it on healthy skin. The herb is used internally by medical herbalists for treating jaundice and gall bladder disease. Its bitterness increases bile flow and it helps to reduce pain from gallstones. However, internal use of the fresh herb is not recommended without consulting a medical herbalist, as it has potentially toxic effects when used in the wrong dose.

What to look for

Celandine grows 20–40 cm (8–16 in) high and 30 cm (12 in) wide. It has bright green, deeply cut leaves with rounded teeth on a hairy stem. The flowers are yellow and resemble buttercups, except that they only have four petals and long, yellow stamens in the centre. The seedpods are long and when ripe contain many tiny, shiny, black seeds. The whole plant exudes a bright orange sap when broken.

Can be mistaken for

Celandine looks like a member of the Cruciferae

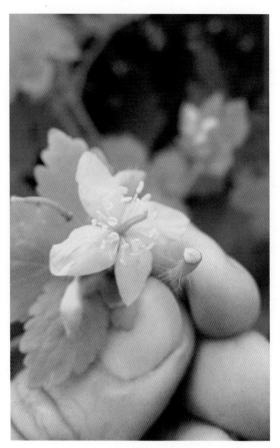

Regularly apply the bright orange sap of greater celandine to warts and verrucas to kill the wart virus.

family because of its four-petalled flowers, although it actually belongs to the poppy family, Papaveraceae. It is not related to lesser celandine or pilewort (see page 50).

Where to look

Celandines are commonly found growing in the shade by old walls and by hedges and on waste ground.

Celandine

When to look for it

Celandine will grow all year round in mild climates. It flowers from May to September.

What to harvest

The whole flowering plant and sap.

What is it good for?

Warts and verrucas

How to use it

Pick a leaf or stem and dab a bit of sap directly onto the wart or verruca on a daily basis. Avoid contact with healthy surrounding skin. The wart will turn brown and then black and should eventually peel off leaving healthy skin underneath. Treat one wart at a time to avoid soreness. The properties may be preserved by making a fresh herb tincture, but this is not as effective as the fresh sap. For internal use in the treatment of jaundice or gallstones, this powerful remedy should only be used under the direction of a medical herbalist.

Cautions

Do not treat warts on the face or genitals with the sap as it might cause scarring or irritation to delicate mucous membranes. For internal use, consult a medical herbalist. Unexplained and obstructive jaundice requires specialist treatment from a qualified medical practitioner.

Combines well with

Dandelion sap (see page 114) for warts and verrucas

Forager's checklist

* ❋ **Perennial herb**
* ❋ **Widely distributed**
* ❋ **Topical wart treatment**
* ❋ **Frequently grows by walls**
* ❋ **Irritant orange sap**
* ❋ **Harvest whole plant when in flower**
* ❋ **Wear gloves to avoid staining skin**
* ❋ **20–40 cm (8–16 in) high and 30 cm (12 in) wide**
* ❋ **Family: Papaveraceae**

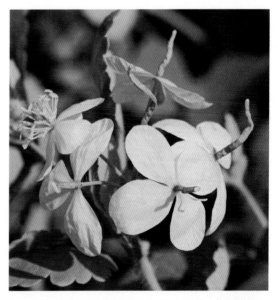

A member of the poppy family, greater celandine flowers are similar in structure to poppies with their four petals.

Waste ground plants

Hypericum perforatum

St John's wort

perforate St John's wort

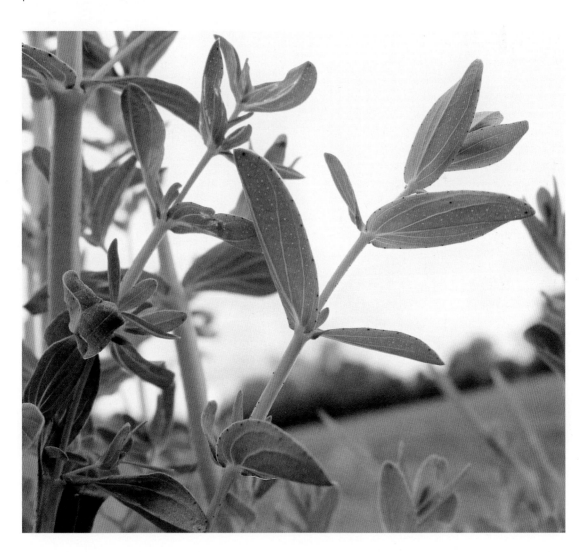

Waste ground plants

Fact and folklore

St John's wort flowers around midsummer, which is where the name comes from, because St John's day is also midsummer's day. The name *Hypericum* comes from the Greek meaning 'over an apparition' because they thought it drove away evil spirits. The yellow flowers exude a red stain in oil, which is used to promote healing in wounds, burns and psoriasis.

The whole plant is well known for its nerve restorative properties and has been shown to be more effective and have fewer side-effects than orthodox medications in the treatment of mild to moderate depression. It is also slightly bitter, helping the liver to excrete depressive toxins. The herb is good for treating viruses, especially ones that have an effect on the central nervous system, such as herpes, chickenpox and shingles. It is also very useful for conditions such as glandular fever, myalgic encephalitis (ME) and chronic fatigue syndrome.

What to look for

A perennial plant that grows 30–60 cm (1–2 ft) high and 30 cm (1 ft) wide, St John's wort is hairless with oval, veined leaves on strong, round stems. When held up to the sun, the leaves appear to be 'perforated', allowing the light to shine through. The stems branch at the top and bear clusters of bright yellow flowers that have five petals and long, yellow stamens with small, yellow, pollen-bearing anthers; on close inspection a hint of red can be seen there.

Can be mistaken for

There are about 17 species of *Hypericum*, including hairy St John's wort (*H. hirsutum*) and bog St John's wort (*H. eloides*). *Perforatum* has a line of dark dots around the margin of the leaves.

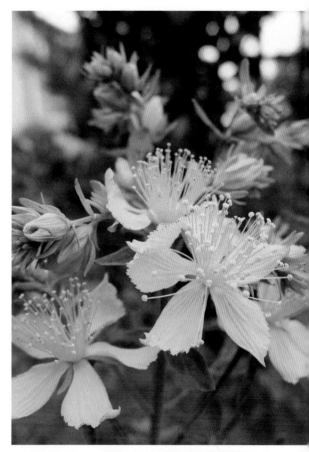

St John's wort flowers leave a red stain when crushed in the fingers and the leaves are perforated with tiny holes.

Where to look

Search for this plant in waste ground and waysides including over-grown footpaths and deserted railway sidings.

When to look for it

St John's wort flowers from June to September.

What to harvest

The whole flowering plant, and the individual flowers.

What is it good for?

Bruises • Burns • Cold sores • Psoriasis • Sunburn • Wounds • Backache • Restless leg syndrome • Anxiety and stress • Chickenpox and shingles • Depression • Neuralgia • Incontinence • Menopause • Premenstrual tension (PMT)

How to use it

Make the whole plant into a fresh herb tincture, which turns a lovely red colour. Dry the herb for making a slightly bitter herbal infusion. Gather the flowers over a number of weeks and add them to a bottle of oil to allow them to infuse and impart their healing properties for the topical treatment of sunburn, burns, bruises, psoriasis, chickenpox, restless leg syndrome and shingles.

Cautions

St John's wort has been shown to increase an enzyme system in the body called cytochrome P450, and this can promote the removal of medications from the body. Ensure you do not take St John's wort if you are taking any prescription medication without first consulting with your doctor and a medical herbalist.

Combines well with

Oat (see page 93) for depression, anxiety and nerve damage or infection
Plantain-infused oil (see page 105) for topical treatment of psoriasis
Wild garlic (see page 41) and elderberry (see page 184) for the treatment of viral illness.

Forager's checklist

❋ **Perennial herb**
❋ **Widely distributed**
❋ **'Perforated' leaves**
❋ **Flowers yield a red oil**
❋ **In flower from June**
❋ **Use whole plant for tinctures**
❋ **Use flowers for infused oil**
❋ **Nerve restorative**
❋ **Antiviral properties**
❋ **30–60 cm (1–2 ft) high and 30 cm (1 ft) wide**
❋ **Family: Hypericaceae/Guttiferae**

St John's wort

Try it in St John's wort-infused oil

This oil is antiseptic and vulnerary (stimulates tissue repair). It can be used for its healing properties as a simple oil or made into a salve either on its own or combined with other infused oils. Pick fresh flowers on a dry, sunny day and pack them into a clean glass jar. Cover the flowers with sunflower oil and screw on the lid. Leave on a sunny windowledge, shaking the jar every few days. Add more flowers as they open, ensuring that the level of oil is kept topped up to keep the flowers submerged. Watch the oil turn red over a few weeks. Strain the oil after a minimum of two weeks. Store in a clean bottle and label. As for all infused oils, it will keep for up to a year. If it smells rancid it is no longer of any use.

Inula helenium

Elecampane

wild sunflower

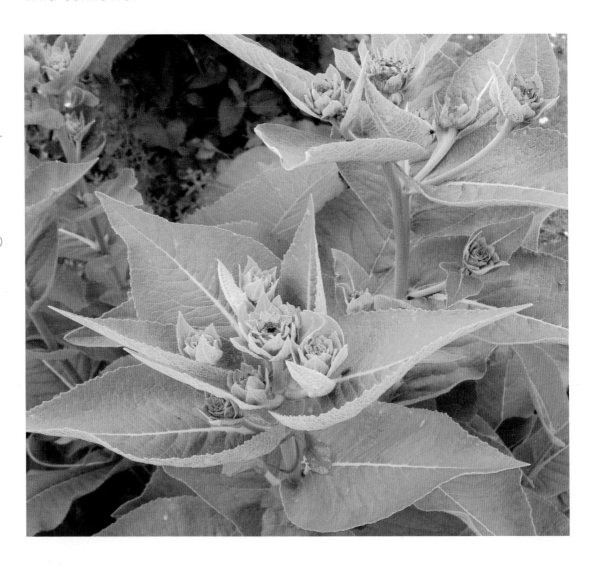

Fact and folklore

Elecampane has been cultivated and used as a medicinal plant since Roman times. The root is highly aromatic, antiseptic and warming and used for the treatment of damp, cold, chesty coughs that are characterized by copious green and yellow phlegm. Its antiseptic drying properties are also useful for relieving mucus of the upper respiratory tract. This is a good remedy for children who seem to have perpetually runny noses, and whose appetites are poor, as its bitter principle will stimulate their appetite and liver and the antiseptic warming properties will reduce bacterial infection and break up thick mucus. It also has bitter properties that make it good for stimulating the digestion and appetite, and especially for indigestion and fullness after meals.

What to look for

Elecampane is a large plant, 1–1.5 m (3–5 ft) high and 60 cm (2 ft) wide. The large, thick roots have an aromatic scent. The leaves are large, usually over 30 cm (1 ft) long, and oval with a pointed end. They are mid-green on top and pale underneath covered with a fine, felty down. The large, yellow, daisy-like flowers form on the top of tall, branching stems and are about 5–8 cm (2–3^1/$_2$ in) across.

Can be mistaken for

The leaves resemble comfrey (see page 76), but elecampane leaves are soft to the touch, with pale, felty undersides, and comfrey leaves are rough and a darker green.

Where to look

Elecampane grows in damp, shady ground alongside canals and rivers, and on over-grown waste ground. It is widespread but not common. Elecampane is also easily cultivated and can make an attractive garden plant.

When to look for it

The leaves begin to grow in April and the plant flowers in July.

What to harvest

The roots in autumn or early spring, from 2–3-year-old plants.

What is it good for?

Asthma • Bronchitis • Catarrh • Coughs • Sinusitis • Sore throat • Indigestion

How to use it

Harvest the root in autumn, when the leaves have mostly died back, by digging round it and collecting a few of the 'runner' roots that are growing out from the main rootball. Replant the main plant. It may be divided into separate plants to propagate it. Use elecampane to make a fresh root tincture. Its properties are also well preserved in a syrup or herbal honey. The root may be chopped and dried for use in decoctions. It can also be candied and eaten as a sweet after meals to improve the digestion.

Cautions

This is a warming and drying herb so is not of use for dry, irritated coughs.

Combines well with

Elderflower (see page 184) and ground ivy (see page 175) for nasal catarrh
Wild thyme (see page 204) for chesty coughs

Elecampane

Waste ground plants

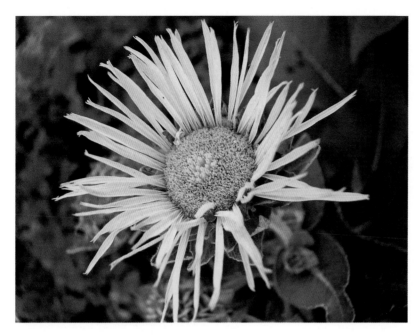

The large, yellow, daisy-like flowers of elecampane show that it is ruled by the sun and has warming properties.

Try it in elecampane honey

This honey treats infections of the upper respiratory tract. Gather the roots and scrub the mud from them. Slice very thinly, put into a jar and cover with honey. Let it infuse for at least a week. The root can be left in the honey. Store the honey in the refrigerator for up to six months. Take for sore throats, sinus congestion and productive coughs, and for indigestion after meals. Children should take 1 teaspoon and adults 1–2 teaspoons, up to four times a day. A piece of the honeyed root can also be chewed and swallowed. Do not give to children under 2 years (see page 35).

Forager's checklist

* Large perennial herb
* Big, yellow, daisy-like flowers
* Warming expectorant
* Root is used
* Harvest in autumn or early spring
* 1–1.5 m (3–5 ft) high and 60 cm (2 ft) wide
* Family: Compositae

Rosa canina

Dog rose

wild rose

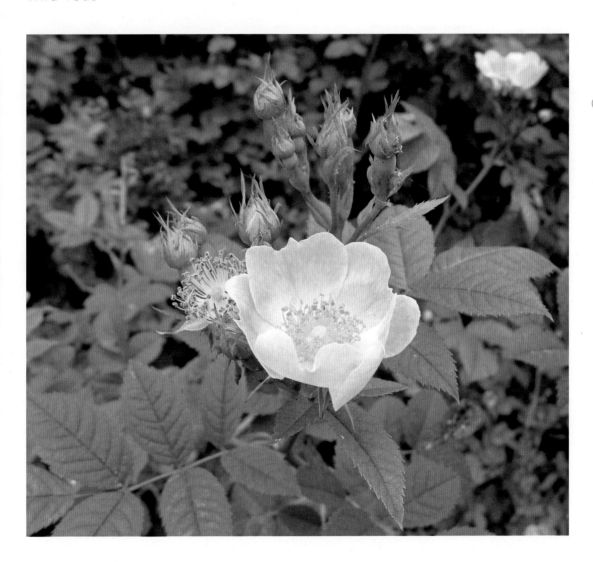

Fact and folklore

The rosary is supposedly so called because in the Middle Ages dried rosehips were used, in place of beads, to count the prayers as they were said. Dog rose has long been used as a food colour in confectionery and desserts, and medicinally the hips are much prized for their high vitamin C content. Traditionally the hips were gathered in large quantities and dried or made into syrups or jellies to keep colds at bay during the winter months. The petals are astringent and can be used for the treatment of diarrhoea, sore mouths and heavy menstrual bleeding. The cooling properties of a petal infusion will help chase away a fever.

What to look for

The dog rose grows to 2 m (6 ft) high and wide, and has horned stems with 5–7 branched, narrowly serrated leaves. The five-petalled flowers vary in colour from pale to deep pink and measure 4–5 cm (1³/4–2 in) across. The blooms can occur singly or in small groups; each flower has many stamens in the centre. The distinctive, bright red, oval fruits, or hips, are 1.5 cm (³/4 in) long.

Can be mistaken for

Of the 14 different species of wild rose, four are varieties of dog rose. The flowers vary in colour and the hips vary in shape, but they are interchangeable medicinally. There is a folk rhyme that helps to identify them:

'On a sultry day, in sunny weather, five brethren were born together
Two had beards and two had none and the other had but half a one.'

This refers to the five sepals of the flower, two of

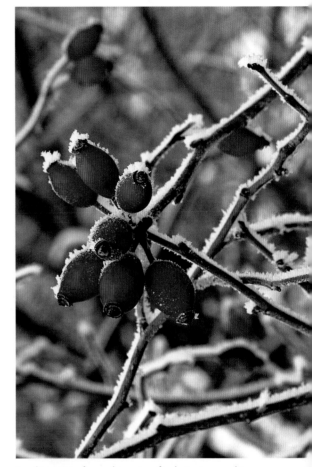

Rosehips are softer and sweeter after being exposed to a frost; however, they may be used before a frost.

which are hairy on both sides, two are smooth, and the last is only hairy on one side.

Where to look

The dog rose is commonly found growing in hedgerows, thickets, at the margins of woodland and on rocky slopes.

When to look for it

The dog rose flowers from May to June. The hips develop in late summer to autumn.

What to harvest

The flowers and hips.

What is it good for?

Acne vulgaris • Acne rosacea • Conjunctivitis • Gums and teeth • Colds • Flu • Bleeding • Exhaustion • Fever • Diarrhoea • Heavy periods

How to use it

Harvest the flower petals when the yellow stamens are bright and fresh and before they turn brown. Use the petals in salads or make into a fresh tincture. Dried petals can be used in infusions for a tea or applied cooled as skin wash for oily skin and the treatment of acne or as an eyewash for conjunctivitis.

Pick the hips when they are red and ripe; they are better after a frost. They contain seeds that are surrounded by many small hairs. These are irritating if ingested and must be removed. If drying hips for infusions, you must split each hip and scrape out the hairs before use. Wear gloves while preparing the hips to avoid the seeds irritating the skin.

Cautions

None.

Combines well with

Shepherd's purse (see page 131) for heavy menstrual bleeding
Elderberry (see page 184) for viral infections
Ground ivy (see page 175) and chamomile (see page 102) as an infusion and use as an eyewash for conjunctivitis

Try it in rosehip syrup

This delicious syrup can be taken in dessertspoon doses or poured onto porridge, fruit salads or pancakes for a rich source of vitamin C. Chop up 500 g (1 lb) rosehips by hand or in a blender, then add them to 1 litre (1³/4 pints) boiling water and bring to the boil. Turn off the heat, cover and leave to infuse for half an hour or so. Strain through a muslin or jelly bag to remove the fine, irritating hairs. Put the liquid on one side.

Put the pulp back in the pan with another 500 ml (17 fl oz) boiling water and bring to the boil. Leave to infuse again, then strain again. Combine all the infused liquid into a clean pan and boil until the volume has reduced by half. Add 500 g (1 lb) sugar and stir until dissolved, then bring up to the boil for five minutes. Bottle in sterilized jars. Label and store in a cool place. Store in the refrigerator after opening. This will keep up to six months but discard if it goes mouldy.

Dog rose

Forager's checklist

※ **Sweet-scented, pink flowers**

※ **Hips are more potent after exposure to frost**

※ **Shrubby hedgerow plant**

※ **Thorny stems**

※ **Hips a rich source of vitamin C**

※ **2 m (6 ft) high and wide**

※ **Family: Rosaceae**

Solidago virgaurea
Golden rod
aaron's rod

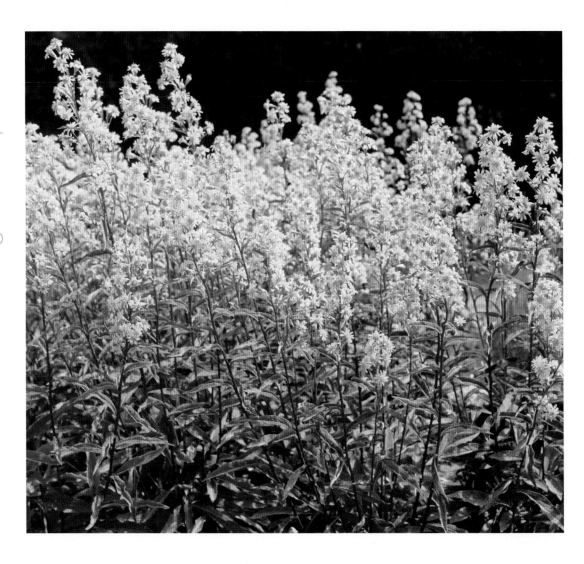

Fact and folklore

Golden rod has a long history of use as a medicine, especially as a diuretic, and there is a record of it being given over a few months to a patient who then passed a number of large stones. The name *Solidago* comes from the Latin meaning to make whole and it was traditionally used as a wound healer. The herb is aromatic and diuretic and used for inflammation and irritation of the urinary system. Its antispasmodic and antiseptic properties make it especially useful for flushing out urinary stones and for treating infection of the urinary system. Its aroma also makes it effective for the treatment of nasal catarrh and congestion, either for chronic conditions such as hayfever or for acute colds. The pollen from golden rod is carried by insects and does not cause hayfever as windborne pollens do.

What to look for

Golden rod is a perennial plant, 30–60 cm (12–24 in) high and 10 cm (4 in) wide. It has upright stems and pointed, finely toothed leaves. The yellow, daisy-like flowers appear from late summer to early autumn.

Can be mistaken for

Often pictured instead is Canadian golden rod (*Solidago canadensis*), which has similar medicinal properties. The flowers are similar to that of ragwort (*Senecio jacobea*), but ragwort's leaves are deeply cut and it has an unpleasant, acrid smell. Its flowers grow at the top of its branched stem. Ragwort is poisonous, so take care not to mistake it for golden rod.

Where to look

Golden rod can be found growing in dry, well-drained soil on heaths and banks and on cliffs.

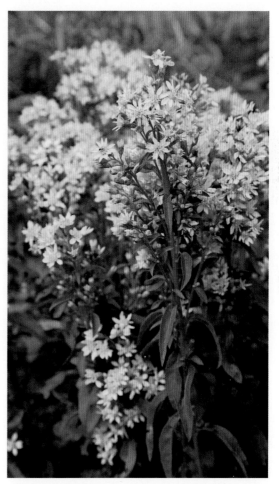

The flowers of golden rod are similar to that of the poisonous ragwort; the leaves, however, are markedly different.

When to look for it

Golden rod grows from April until October and flowers from July to September.

What to harvest

The whole flowering plant.

Golden rod

What is it good for?

Catarrh • Colds • Hayfever • Cystitis • Kidney stones

How to use it

Harvest the whole flowering herb and dry it for use in herbal infusions for urinary problems, to increase urine flow. Regular infusions will help to reduce the risk of kidney stones developing if there is a predisposition to them. Taken hot during colds, it will help to dry up a runny nose. Make a tincture with the fresh or dried herb for use alone, or combine in a mix with other herbs, for treatment of chronic nasal catarrh, hayfever or colds.

Cautions

Do not use in combination with orthodox diuretics.

Combines well with

Cramp bark (see page 187) and dandelion leaf (see page 114) for urinary stones
Wild thyme (see page 204) and plantain (see page 105) for urinary infections

Try it for flushing out urinary stones

Urinary stones are recurrent. If you are unlucky enough to develop them once, you have an increased chance of getting them again. The two most common types of stone are: calcium oxalate stones that form because the kidney is not flushing out calcium efficiently; and struviate stones that develop as a result of recurrent urine infections. There are a few things you can do to significantly reduce the risk of recurrence:

- Increase your fluid intake to at least 2 litres (3^{1}/$_{2}$ pints) a day

Forager's checklist

❋ **Two main varieties**
❋ **Perennial plant**
❋ **Widely distributed**
❋ **Urinary tonic**
❋ **Harvest the flowering plant**
❋ **Flowers from July to September**
❋ **Use the dried plant for infusion**
❋ **30–60 cm (12–24 in) high and 10 cm (3 in) wide**
❋ **Family: Compositae**

- Magnesium reduces the risk, so increase your intake of magnesium-rich foods
- Eat more fruit and vegetables
- Drink less tea and coffee
- Reduce oxalate foods such as spinach, rhubarb, chocolate and strawberries
- Reduce salt consumption
- Maintain a good calcium intake
- Drink plenty of diuretic herbal teas, such as golden rod, couch grass, dandelion leaf and nettle

Stellaria media

Chickweed

starweed

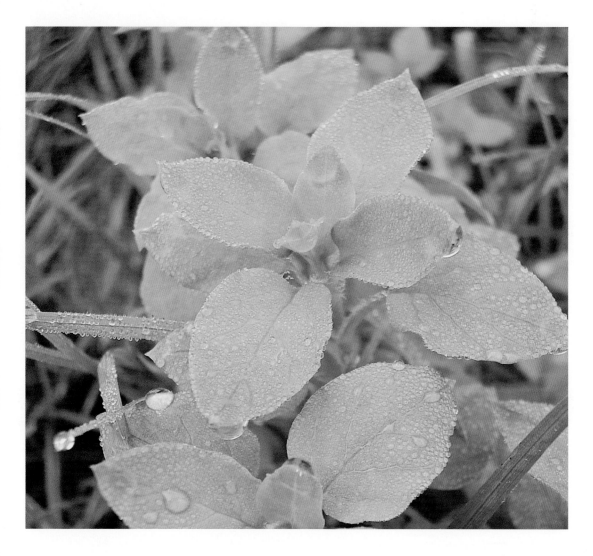

Fact and folklore

The name *Stellaria* comes from the Latin for 'star', which explains the common name starweed. Chickweed water was traditionally thought to be a remedy for weight loss. Chickweed is often fed to caged birds, and may be eaten either as a salad vegetable or cooked. It is rich in minerals and trace elements, particularly iron, magnesium, manganese, silicon and zinc. The juice of the fresh herb relieves itching of the skin, and it is used internally and externally for the treatment of hot, irritated skin conditions. It helps to eliminate toxins via the urinary system and by gently stimulating bowel function.

What to look for

Chickweed is a low-growing, clump-forming annual, 10–40 cm (4–16 in) high and wide. It has bright, fresh green, oval, pointed leaves. Small, white, star-like flowers each have five petals that are almost divided to their base. There is a single line of hairs on the stem.

Can be mistaken for

There are about 100 different members of the Caryophyllaceae family. The various chickweeds and stitchworts have similar medicinal properties. Mouse-ears (*Cerastium* spp.) have similar flowers and petal structure, but unlike chickweed, their leaves and stems are uniformly hairy.

Where to look

Chickweed grows in most soils on waste ground and footpaths. It can also be found under trees, and in meadows and field margins.

When to look for it

It grows and flowers from March to November.

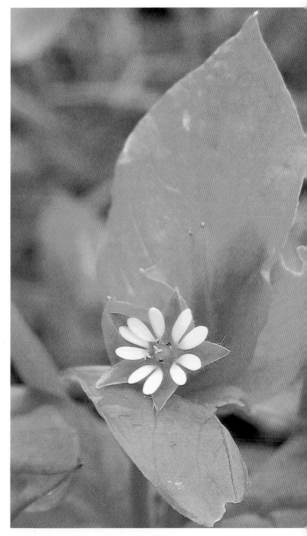

The petals of chickweed's star-like flowers are deeply divided to their base so they look like two petals, rather than one.

What to harvest

The whole plant.

What is it good for?

Boils • Conjunctivitis • Eczema • Psoriasis •
Anaemia • Chickenpox and shingles • Cystitis

How to use it

Pick the fresh plant and pulverize it in a little water.
Use the resulting juice as a skin lotion for itching and
inflamed skin, or as an eyewash for irritated eyes up
to six times a day. Freeze any excess juice in ice-cube
trays and use as required. Bruise the fresh herb and
use as a drawing poultice for boils and abscesses.
Replace every few hours. Make an infused oil from
some of the fresh herb that has been wilted overnight
and use for itching skin conditions. Use the dry herb as
an infusion for its cleansing properties for skin disease
and rheumatic conditions. Make a fresh herb tincture
for internal use.

Cautions

Do not take chickweed if you have irritation or
bleeding of the stomach or intestines as chickweed
may aggravate this condition.

Combines well with

Chamomile (see page 102) and plantain (see page
105) in a salve for eczema, skin rashes and psoriasis
Nettle (see page 155) and meadowsweet (see page
169) for rheumatic disease

Try it in chickweed salve

Use this salve to preserve the anti-itch and anti-
inflammatory properties of chickweed. It also has the
added benefit of moisturizing oils and a water-
resistant barrier of beeswax for dry skin conditions.
First make an infused oil. Gather a large quantity of
fresh chickweed and leave it to wilt overnight. Place half
in a glass bowl and set it over a pan of water on the
cooker, so that the base of the bowl sits in the water.
Bring the water up to a gentle simmer. Pour the
sunflower oil over the chickweed to just cover. Leave to
infuse for two hours. Then strain the herb and oil,
pressing out all the oil. Put the remaining wilted herb
in the bowl, pour the same oil over it and repeat the
process. To make 25 g (1oz) of soft set salve, put 25 ml
(1 fl oz) infused oil in a pan and grate in 5 g ($^1/4$ oz)
beeswax. When it has melted, check the consistency
dipping in a cold teaspoon. The salve will quickly set.
Add more beeswax if you require a harder salve. Pour
into a pot and leave to set. It will keep up to a year. It
combines well with chamomile-infused oil when made
into a salve to increase its anti-inflammatory properties.
Use equal amounts of chamomile and chickweed-
infused oils and then add the beeswax.

Forager's checklist

* **Abundant annual weed**
* **Best harvested in early summer for lush foliage**
* **Widely distributed**
* **Tiny, star-like, white flowers**
* **Many different varieties**
* **Anti-itching**
* **Fresh herb preparations for topical use**
* **Freeze the juice in ice-cube trays**
* **10–40 cm (4–16 in) high and wide**
* **Family: Caryophyllaceae**

Chickweed

Tussilago farfara

Coltsfoot

coughwort, horsehoof

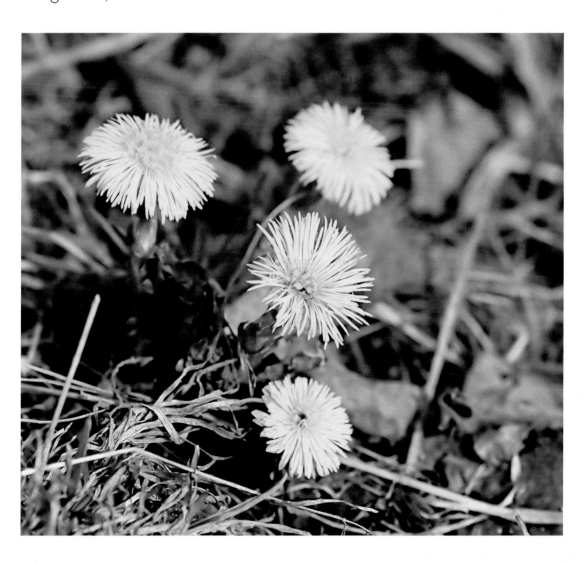

Fact and folklore

Tussilago means 'cough dispeller', and coltsfoot has long been used as an anti-cough remedy. The common name arose because the leaf shape was thought to resemble a colt's foot. The leaves are often included in herbal smoking mixes, which were traditionally thought to be beneficial for the treatment of bronchitis and asthma. The herb is now used internally for the treatment of tickly, dry coughs; it works by soothing the irritated airways, allowing the patient to get a good night's sleep. The leaves and flowers, however, contain small amounts of pyrollizidine alkaloids, like those found in comfrey but at much lower concentrations. These are accumulative over time in the body and may have potentially liver-damaging effects. Reports of problems on humans are rare and research has involved experiments on rats. However, be aware of the potential risks if using coltsfoot. It is only recommended for short-term use, a few weeks a year.

What to look for

Coltsfoot grows up to 25 cm (10 in) high, and is usually distributed over a wide area. The flowers appear before the leaves, each on a single stem that has reddish, scale-like leaflets and is covered with a fine, cobweb-like down. The flower is yellow with multiple fine petals at its margin, and the centre consists of many tiny florets. The leaves emerge when the flowers have gone to seed. They are stalked and round with slightly angled edges, with a heart-shaped base where the leaf is attached to the stem. The underside is covered with fine, white hair. When the flowers go to seed they form a white, downy ball that gets dispersed on the slightest breeze, carrying the seed far afield.

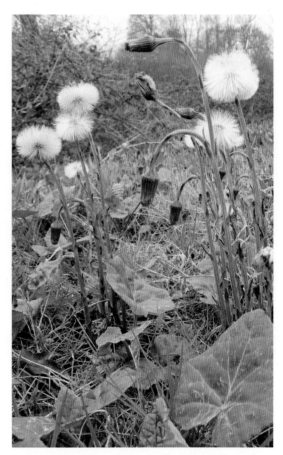

The leaves of coltsfoot emerge after the plant has flowered and gone to seed.

Coltsfoot

Can be mistaken for

The leaves of butterbur (*Petasites hybridus*) are similar, but generally larger, more rounded and finely toothed. It, too, flowers before the leaves appear, but the flowers are significantly different.

Where to look

Coltsfoot grows in rough waste ground and poor soils.

Waste ground plants

When to look for it
It flowers in February and March, and the leaves grow from April to September.

What to harvest
The flowers and leaves.

What is it good for?
Asthma • Bronchitis • Coughs

How to use it
Gather the leaves for use in infusions. The tincture may be made with fresh or dry herb and used in combinations for the treatment of tickly coughs. Gather the flowers for use in a syrup or dry for use in infusions.

Cautions
Coltsfoot leaf has been shown to contain small amounts of potentially liver-damaging compounds. Use it only for short periods (no more than two weeks). Do not use in pregnancy or for treating young children.

Combines well with
Mallow (see page 64) for dry coughs
Mullein (see page 158) and wild thyme (see page 204) for asthma

Try it in coltsfoot flower syrup
Infuse 25 g (1 oz) coltsfoot flowers in 600 ml (1 pint) water by simmering them in a pan for ten minutes. Strain out the flowers and reduce the infusion, by simmering, to a third of its volume. For every 200 ml (7 fl oz) of liquid, add 400 ml (14 fl oz) honey or 150 g (5 oz) sugar. Stir well until dissolved, then bottle and

Forager's checklist
❋ **Perennial herb**
❋ **Widely distributed**
❋ **Flowers appear before the leaves**
❋ **Grows in poor soil**
❋ **Take for short periods only**
❋ **25 cm (10 in) high and 30 cm (12 in) wide**
❋ **Family: Compositae**

label. Take 1–2 teaspoons, every two hours for acute tickly coughs, or four times a day for chronic coughs. Do not use for longer than two weeks.

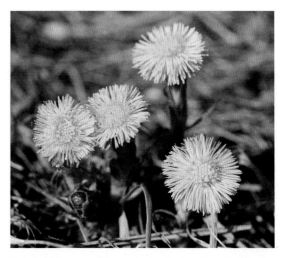

Coltsfoot flowers and leaves can be used medicinally; the flowers traditionally are made into syrup.

Urtica dioica

Nettle

stinging nettle

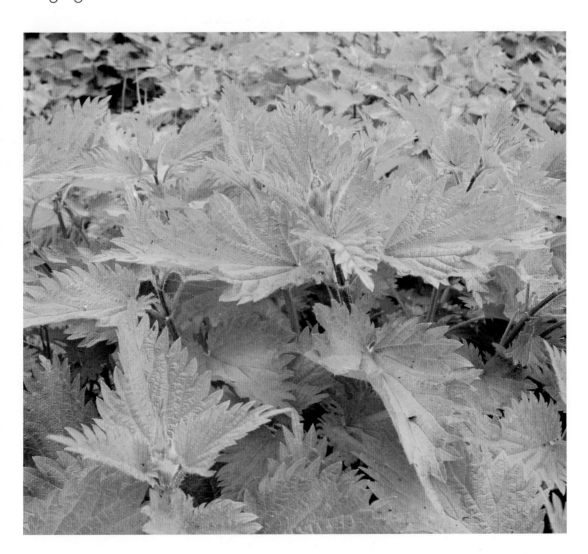

Waste ground plants

Fact and folklore

Nettles have a multitude of properties, not only medicinal, and have been used for fabric and fibres, dyes, food and paper. The Romans used their sting to stimulate the circulation in their extremities when faced with the cold weather in Britain. They are extremely nutritious, being rich in vitamins A and C, iron, magnesium, calcium, chromium, zinc, potassium, phosphorus and silicon. They are anti-allergenic and have been shown to reduce histamine production, so are good for hayfever and wet eczema.

Nettles are reputed to reduce blood-sugar levels. Their sting has been shown to reduce pain in arthritic joints – taken internally they remove toxins and acid from the joints and eliminate it in the urine. They have astringent properties and with their iron content are good for anaemia and bleeding. Use them at the end of pregnancy and after labour for their toning and nutritional benefits. They are also reputed to increase breast milk. The roots have been shown to be beneficial for the symptoms of prostate disease. The seeds are strengthening and restorative for the adrenal glands. The seeds can also be used to make a hair rinse to tone the scalp.

What to look for

The nettle is a perennial plant that grows from multiple points on a shallow, branching root system, to 1.2 m (4 ft) tall, over wide areas. The roots are yellow. The whole plant is covered with fine, but visible, stinging hairs. The stem is square, and the deeply serrated leaves are heart-shaped at the base and pointed at the top. The flowers and seeds are borne on long, drooping stems from the stem and leaf axils; the plants bear either male (barren) or female (seed-producing) flowers.

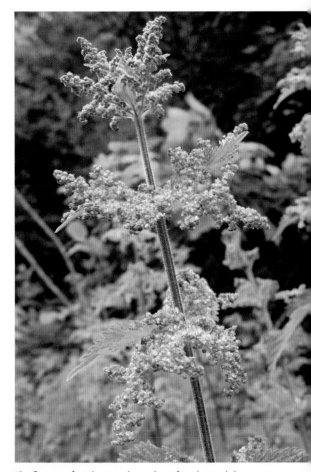

The flowers of nettles may be male or female, each borne on different plants. The female flower produces seeds, which have medicinal properties.

Can be mistaken for

Deadnettles (*Lamium* spp.), motherwort (*Leonurus cardiaca*) and yellow archangel (*Lamiastrum galeobdolon*) look similar, but the nettle's stinging abilities are its unmistakable feature. The small nettle (*Urtica urens*) is interchangeable with the common nettle.

Where to look

It is said that nettles only grow in fertile earth. They can be found growing prolifically in hedgerows, wood margins, waste ground, meadows, gardens and roadsides.

When to look for it

Nettles start growing in March and continue until hard winter frosts.

What to harvest

The whole plant and its roots.

What is it good for?

Eczema • Arthritis • Gout • Osteoporosis • Hayfever • Anaemia • Bleeding • Exhaustion • Allergies • Prostate problems • Heavy periods

How to use it

Pick the young herb and dry it in bundles for use in infusions – nettle is a pleasant-tasting tea that can be drunk daily. Make the fresh herb tincture for combination with other herbs. Harvest the root and make fresh root tincture. Alternatively, strip the dried seeds from the stem and rub through a fine sieve to remove the sting. Take a dessertspoon once a day in yogurt or in food to nourish and strengthen the adrenal glands.

Cautions

Do not use during early pregnancy. Nettles are hot by nature, so do not take for hot and dry conditions or for example in eczema when the skin is hot and dry to the touch, as they may aggravate the condition. Do not use leaves after flowering as they can accumulate irritating constituents.

Forager's checklist

* **Invasive perennial plant**
* **Stinging hairs**
* **Common in all ground**
* **Widely distributed**
* **Rich in nutrients**
* **Harvest plants when young and fresh**
* **Wear gloves to protect hands**
* **Anti-allergenic**
* **1.2 m (4 ft) high**
* **Family: Urticaceae**

Nettle

Combines well with

Plantain (see page 105) for allergies
Meadowsweet (see page 169) for arthritis

Try it in nettle soup

Sauté a chopped onion in a little oil. Add a peeled, chopped potato and a chopped clove of garlic. Add 2 large handfuls of young, fresh nettle tops. Stir for a few minutes and add boiling water to cover the nettles by a few centimetres. Add 1 teaspoon bouillon or chicken stock powder. Put the lid on and simmer for 25 minutes until the potato is soft. Add 1 handful of wild garlic leaves (see page 41) for the last five minutes (optional). Blend the soup and serve.

Verbascum thapsus

Mullein

candlewick, torches

Fact and folklore

Mullein comes from the Latin word *mollis*, meaning 'soft'. Its other common names derive from its flammable properties and use as kindling and as a torchlight when dipped in tallow. The large, soft leaves were used as a shoe liner by country people to keep their feet warm in winter. Mullein is used as a soothing remedy for all kinds of lung irritations. It will also break up thick catarrh in the lungs and nose, enabling its expulsion from the body. It is also gently sedating, making it useful for spasmodic coughs, especially at night in children. The infused oil from the flowers is good for ear irritation and infections such as glue ear, and to loosen earwax.

What to look for

Mullein is a biennal plant that (apart from the flowers) is covered in dense, soft fur, giving it a whitish, frosted appearance; underneath it is pale green. In the first year, the large, soft, round-ended leaves, which resemble rabbits' ears, form a large basal rosette 20–60 cm (8–24 in) wide. In the second year, one thick, straight stem grows up to 2 m (6 ft). It is covered in yellow, five-petalled flowers. Later in the season, the main stem may form branches, each branch bearing more flowers.

Can be mistaken for

In its first year, the basal rosette may resemble that of a foxglove (*Digitalis purpurea*), which is poisonous. The leaves of mullein are rounded at the ends and covered in a dense, fine down whereas foxglove leaves are pointed and not nearly as densely covered with hairs. In the second year, both have a similar flower spike, but foxglove flowers are trumpet-shaped with spotted centres and of different colours.

Mullein

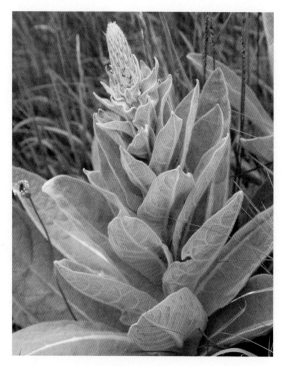

The flowering stalk of mullein may grow up to 2 m (6 ft) tall. It emerges in the second year of growth.

Where to look

Grows on grass verges, waste ground and hedge banks.

When to look for it

The basal leaf rosette appears in the first year, from June, and remains throughout winter. In the second year, it flowers in June and August.

What to harvest

The leaves and flowers.

What is it good for?

Asthma • Bronchitis • Catarrh • Coughs • Earache

How to use it

Gather the leaves and make a fresh herb tincture for use in cough mixtures. Use a fine strainer to remove the fine hairs, which may irritate, despite the plant's soothing properties. Dry the leaves for use in herbal infusions. Gather the flowers in the second year and make a fresh tincture, or make an infused oil for external use as eardrops.

Cautions

Whooping cough is a notifiable disease; you must inform your doctor if you suspect this infection. Do not use in ears if there is a suspected or confirmed perforated eardrum.

Combines well with

Wild thyme (see page 204) and plantain (see page 105) for asthma and coughs
Infused oil of chamomile (see page 102) for earache and auricular eczema

Try it in mullein earache oil

Gather mullein flowers, over a few weeks if necessary. Place them in a glass jar and pour sunflower or grapeseed oil over them. Screw on the lid and leave the jar on a sunny windowledge, adding more flowers as you harvest them. Keep them submerged in oil. After two to four weeks, strain out the flowers and bottle the oil.

Make the earache oil, as required, by mixing infused oil of chamomile and mullein oil. Add a small clove of garlic, broken in half, and leave to infuse overnight before removing. Use 4 drops every two hours for acute ear complaints such as an infection or deafness from catarrh. Omit the garlic if using for eczema around the ears.

Forager's checklist

* **Tall-stemmed biennial herb**
* **Widely distributed**
* **Large, soft, downy leaves**
* **Soothing respiratory remedy**
* **Roadside and waste ground plant**
* **Harvest leaves in the first year or early part of the second**
* **Harvest flowers in the second year**
* **Beware confusing with foxgloves**
* **2 m (6 ft) high**
* **Family: Scrophulariaceae**

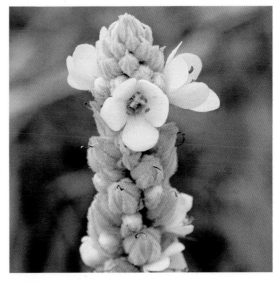

Gather the flowers of mullein and collect them in a jar of oil, leaving it in the sun to infuse.

Verbena officinalis

Vervain

herb of grace

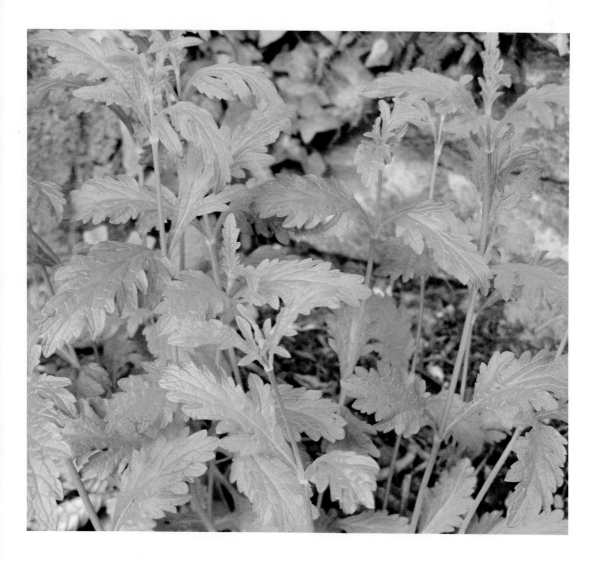

Fact and folklore

Vervain is well known in France, where it is a popular herbal tea. It is a graceful plant producing slender branches with tiny, pinky-white flowers dotted along them. They are said to resemble the nerves and the signals travelling along them. Vervain is known as a nervous system restorative and gentle relaxant used for tension and anxiety. It is also slightly bitter, making it good for digestive problems, especially those associated with nerves and tension, particularly constipation.

The plant's restorative properties are useful for convalescence during and after illness when it will stimulate the appetite and digestion and rebuild a depressed nervous system weakened by illness. It is valuable for depression and low mood to lift the spirits and rejuvenate the system. It has a reputation for female complaints, the bitter action helping the liver with hormone metabolism, calming the nerves and easing mood swings.

What to look for

Vervain is a clump-forming perennial plant. The leaves, which appear in spring, are elongated and deeply cut at the top with round, toothed edges. The numerous long stems that grow out of the clump are rectangular and branching at the top. Some stalkless leaves grow at the base of the stem. Tiny lilac or pinky-white flowers grow directly from the stem, opening gradually up the stem as it grows. There are cultivated ornamental vervains with purple flowers that are not interchangeable medicinally.

Can be mistaken for

Mints (*Mentha* spp.) have a similar growing habit, but vervain is not scented.

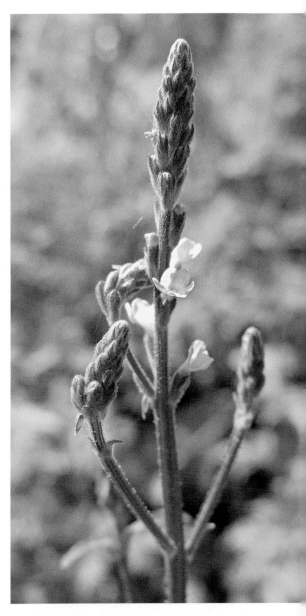

The flowering stems of vervain grow to long lengths and the flowers emerge as they grow in ones and twos.

Where to look
Vervain grows on rough and waste ground.

When to look for it
The leaves begin to grow in April and it flowers from July until September.

What to harvest
The whole plant, just before it flowers.

What is it good for?
Cold sores • Anxiety and stress • Depression • Exhaustion • Insomnia • Constipation • Menopause • Premenstrual tension (PMT)

How to use it
Harvest the whole herb before it flowers and dry for use in infusions. Make a fresh herb tincture, which preserves all of its properties. Take 10 ml (2 teaspoons) of tincture as a single dose to relax constipated bowels.

Cautions
Do not use during pregnancy. Do not stop taking any antidepressants prescribed by your doctor without consulting him or her first.

Combines well with
Oat (see page 93) for convalescence and depression

Try it in vervain flower essence
Flower remedies were originally created by Dr Edward Bach in the 1930s. He initially trained as a doctor and worked as a surgeon, but felt that emotional issues were largely ignored in orthodox medicine and so he investigated the emotional rebalancing effects of flowers. This flower remedy is for highly energetic

Vervain

Forager's checklist
* ❋ Self-seeding perennial
* ❋ Thin, branching stems
* ❋ Delicate, pinky-white flowers
* ❋ Likes well-drained soil in full sun
* ❋ Bitter nervous system tonic
* ❋ Use the whole herb
* ❋ Harvest just before flowering
* ❋ 60–120 cm (2–4 ft) high and 30 cm (1 ft) wide
* ❋ Family: Verbenaceae

people who drive themselves relentlessly, living on nervous energy, encouraging others to follow their lead. This may cause them to become exhausted, and they often suffer nervous collapse. Vervain helps them to use their energy and enthusiasm in a more natural, gentle manner that doesn't alienate others or exhaust themselves. Gather the flowering tips of the plant on a sunny day and float them in a small bowl containing 25 ml (1 fl oz) spring water. Leave this in the sun near the original plant for a few hours to allow the flowers to impart their energy into the water. Use a stem of the plant to lift out the flowers. Pour the water into a 50 ml (2 fl oz) dropper bottle and add 25 ml (1 fl oz) brandy to preserve it for up to three years. Take 4 drops in a little water as required, up to three times a day, or add it into a tincture mix. Alternatively, dilute it into a dosage bottle of 4 drops to 20 ml (3/4 fl oz) of spring water to carry around, and take 4 drops directly onto the tongue as required.

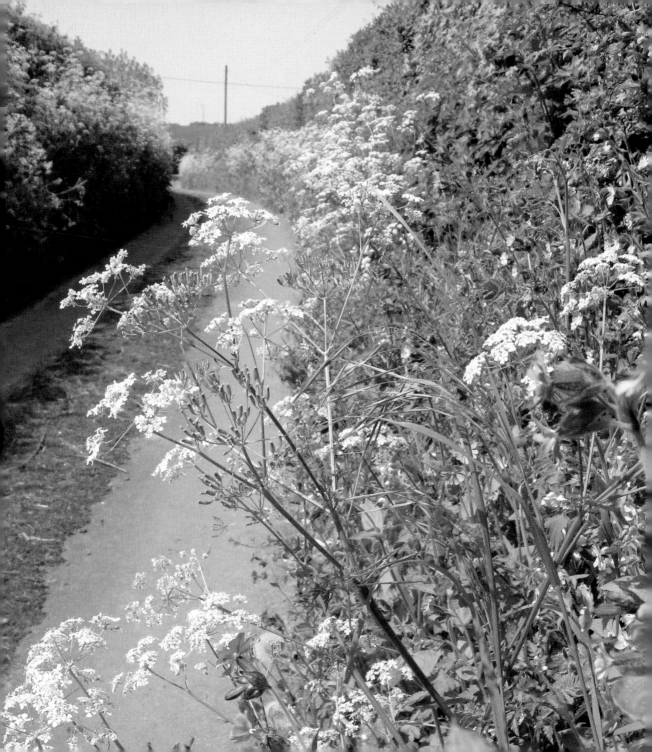

HEDGEROW PLANTS

Hedgerows are a great source of many healing plants, since they are often untouched for many years, and those that are maintained thrive from the annual trimming. Healing herbs such as hawthorn, elder and cramp bark help to form the main structure of the hedge. These shrubby plants also provide a protective screen and climbing frame for the smaller herbs that flourish at their base.

Crataegus monogyna

Hawthorn

bread and cheese, may blossom

Hedgerow plants

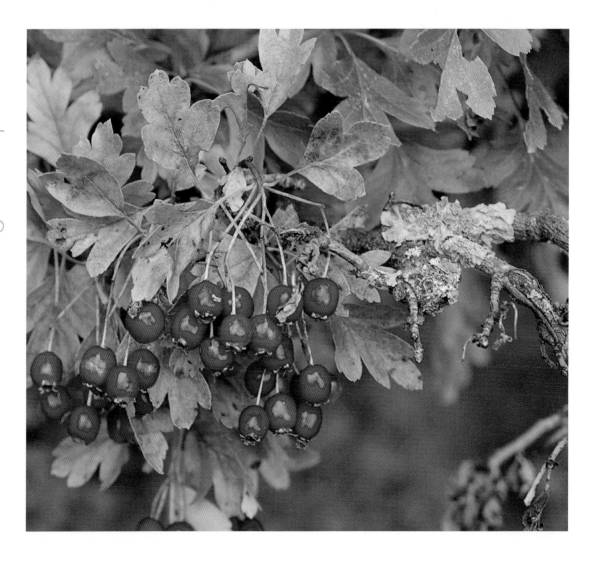

Fact and folklore

It is considered unlucky to bring hawthorn blossom into the house as it is said to smell like death and resemble the stench of the great plague of London, but it is a true sign of spring and the summer to come. In former times, country children knew hawthorn as 'bread and cheese' and often ate the tender young shoots and buds – they are tasty added to salads and sandwiches.

Hawthorn is the prime cardiac tonic used for most heart conditions to strengthen and restore the blood vessels and heart muscle. It is rich in flavonoids that help to reduce arterial stiffening and fatty deposits, improving general blood vessel health and reducing blood pressure. It is also reputed to strengthen the beat and muscle of the heart. The flowers and berries have similar actions, but the berries are often considered to be more useful in lowering blood pressure.

What to look for

Hawthorn is a thorny shrub or small tree that varies in height depending on its location, but can reach 5 m (16 ft). It often grows in hedgerows. The leaves have 5–7 lobes, and white flowers with five petals and many stamens with tiny, yellow anthers are borne in clusters. These develop into bunches of red berries each with one seed (the meaning of *monogyna*).

Can be mistaken for

The smooth-leaved or midland hawthorn (*Crataegus laevigata*) is interchangeable medicinally with *C. monogyna*.

Where to look

It grows in hedgerows, scrubby ground, copses and wood margins.

When to look for it

Hawthorn flowers in May and bears fruit in September.

What to harvest

The flowering stems, including the young leaves and green stalks, the flowers and the berries.

What is it good for?

Atherosclerosis • Chilblains • High cholesterol • High blood pressure

How to use it

Pick the flowering stems to make a fresh herb tincture, or dry the flowers for an infusion to be drunk daily. Harvest the berries for a fresh tincture, which can be combined with the flower-top tincture made earlier in the year to gain the benefits of both parts of the plant. Dry the berries for decoction. The berries make a good tonic wine – take a small glassful every day.

Cautions

Do not use in combination with orthodox cardiac drugs without consultation, as it can increase their effects. If treating high blood pressure, it is advisable to do so with the assistance of a registered medical herbalist and your doctor. Be cautious with hawthorn in cases of low blood pressure, as it may cause it to become even lower.

Combines well with

Lime (see page 56), yarrow (see page 84), cramp bark (see page 187) and mistletoe (see page 59) for high blood pressure

Cramp bark (see page 187) and yarrow (see page 84) for poor circulation and intermittent claudication

Hawthorn

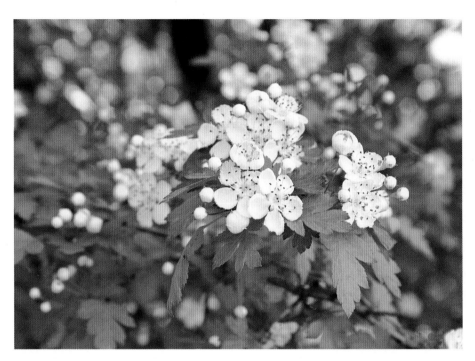

The buds of the flowers and leaves were often eaten by children in the past; they have a delicate pleasant flavour.

Try it in hawthorn berry wine

Put 2.5 litres (4 pints) crushed hawthorn berries into a large pan or bucket and pour over 4.5 litres (1 gallon) of boiling water. Crush and add one campden tablet and stir in 1.25 kg (2^1/$_2$ lb) sugar until it has dissolved. Chop 175 g (6 oz) sultanas and add them to the pan. Put the lid on and leave for 24 hours. Put 1 sachet wine yeast in a small glass of warm water with 1 teaspoon sugar, and leave in a warm place for a few hours. Stir into the must. Leave for two days. Strain into a demijohn, fit an airlock and leave in a warm place until fermentation is finished. Strain into a second demijohn and fit the airlock again. Leave to settle for 8–12 weeks. Have a glass of it to taste and bottle the rest into sterilized bottles. Leave for at least six months to mature.

Forager's checklist

* **Deciduous shrub or tree**
* **Common hedgerow plant**
* **Widely distributed**
* **White blossom in May**
* **Cardinal heart tonic**
* **Rich in blood vessel restorative compounds**
* **2–5 m (6–16 ft) high**
* **Family: Rosaceae**

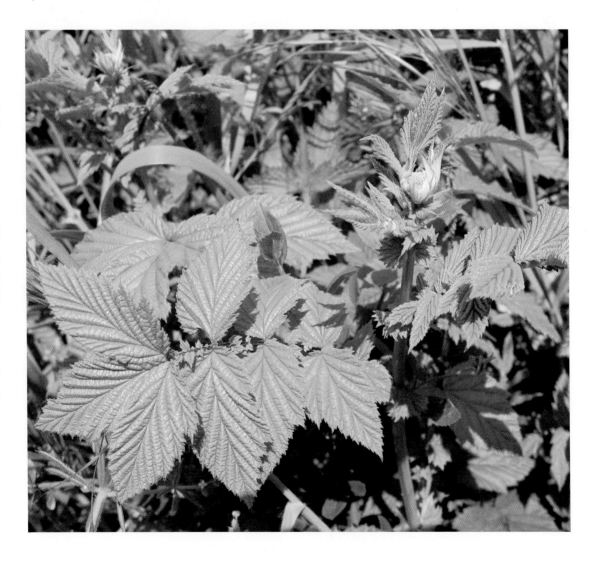

Filipendula ulmaria

Meadowsweet

queen of the meadow

Fact and folklore

Aspirin was named after the former botanical name for meadowsweet, *Spiraea.* Meadowsweet contains salicylate, which is similar to the anti-inflammatory salicylic acid in aspirin. It has a long history of use as a medicine, as a flavouring for mead and as a strewing herb and as stuffing for straw mattresses. One of the traditional medicinal uses involved steeping it in wine and drinking it to drive out fever and make the heart merry. Despite having similar compounds to the stomach-irritating aspirin, meadowsweet has been shown to reduce irritation and inflammation in the stomach. It is used for heartburn, indigestion, gastritis and ulceration. The anti-inflammatory effects also help with joint pain from arthritis.

What to look for

Meadowsweet is a perennial plant, 60–120 cm (2–4 ft) high, with finely toothed leaves growing on long, red-hued stalks. They reduce in number up the flower stem, which is round and branched at the top, bearing a frothy bunch of creamy, pleasantly sharp-scented flowers. Each tiny floret has five petals and comparatively long stamens bearing lots of creamy pollen. The leaves have a more astringent scent.

Can be mistaken for

Dropwort (*Filipendula vulgaris*) is similar, but the leaves are very narrow and deeply cut.

Where to look

Meadowsweet grows in damp ground and partial shade, beside streams and in damp hedgerows.

When to look for it

Look for meadowsweet when the leaves start to

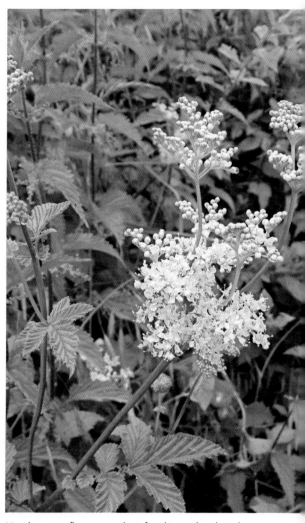

Meadowsweet flowers may be infused into oil and used topically for joint and muscle aches and pains.

appear from April; it flowers in July and August.

What to harvest

The whole flowering plant.

What is it good for?
Acne rosacea • Cold sores • Arthritis • Gout • Sprains and strains • Heartburn • Indigestion

How to use it
Pick meadowsweet and use fresh or dry for infusions. Make a tincture with the fresh herb; this is an effective way to preserve its qualities and ensure regular doses, if the tea is found unpalatable or difficult to adhere to. Make an infused oil of the whole plant for topical use on painful joints and cold sores or as an ointment or liniment.

Cautions
Do not take meadowsweet internally in combination with anticoagulants, including aspirin, as it could potentially increase the effects of these blood-thinning compounds.

Combines well with
Chamomile (see page 102) and mallow (see page 64) for heartburn, gastritis and gastric ulcer
Nettle (see page 155) for arthritis and gout

Try it in meadowsweet and horseradish salve
This salve will provide the anti-inflammatory properties of the salicylates found in meadowsweet and the warming, circulatory-stimulating properties of horseradish, to relieve the stiffness in arthritic joints and strained or aching muscles. You will need some fresh meadowsweet that has been wilted for a few hours. Infuse the meadowsweet for two hours in sunflower or grapeseed oil together with a 2.5 cm (1 in) piece of fresh horseradish root (see page 122), peeled and sliced, per 100 ml (3 1/2 fl oz) of oil. Then roughly strain it and use the same oil and fresh meadowsweet herb, this time omitting the horseradish. Infuse for a further two hours. To make 25 g (1 oz) of soft set salve, strain the oil and return 25 ml (1 fl oz) to a pan with 5 g (1/4 oz) grated beeswax. Check the setting consistency with a cold spoon, adding more beeswax as required, for a harder setting salve. Pour into jars when the desired setting consistency has been reached. Massage into aching joints and limbs up to three times a day. This will keep for up to one year. If it smells rancid, discard it and make a fresh batch. More horseradish may be used if desired. The salve should create a gentle, warm sensation when applied. Different people vary in their sensitivity to the circulatory effects of horseradish.

Forager's checklist
* ❋ **Perennial herb**
* ❋ **Widely distributed**
* ❋ **Grows in damp hedges and beside streams**
* ❋ **Sweet-scented, delicate creamy flowers**
* ❋ **Harvest the whole flowering plant**
* ❋ **Flowers in July and August**
* ❋ **Antacid digestive healer**
* ❋ **Anti-inflammatory properties**
* ❋ **60–120 cm (2–4 ft) high and 30 cm (1 ft) wide**
* ❋ **Family: Rosaceae**

Meadowsweet

Galium aparine
Cleavers
clivers, sticky willy, goose grass

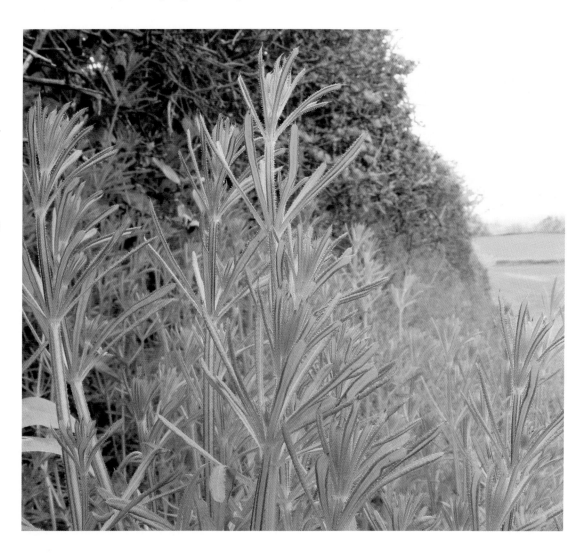

Fact and folklore

Cleavers is among the first spring plants to grow and has an ancient reputation as a spring cleansing tonic. The 2nd-century Greek herbalist Galen said it would make even fat folk lean. Its common names come from its clingy nature – it has hooked stems and leaves to enable it to climb up other plants. The plant has been used by shepherds as a crude sieve for milk to filter out hairs and dirt. The seeds, roasted and ground, were traditionally used as a coffee substitute. The roots are red and yield a red dye, and they were reputed to dissolve and soften kidney stones.

It is used as a lymphatic cleanser in the treatment of skin disease and for swollen glands. Its diuretic properties flush out accumulated wastes and bacteria from and via the urinary tract. It is a cooling remedy and can be used for hot, inflamed skin and joint disease and for urinary infections and stones. It is also used externally to promote healing in skin sores.

What to look for

Cleavers can grow over a large area, and can reach a height of 1.5 m (5 ft). It has quadrangular, hooked, climbing stems with 5–7 leaves forming a whorl around the stem at regular intervals. The flowers are small and white. The seeds are small, green, sticky balls, often found in the coats of pets and children after walks.

Can be mistaken for

Sweet woodruff (*Galium odoratum*) is a much more compact plant, growing closer to the ground, with eight leaves forming each whorl; the leaves are pointed rather than rounded with spiked tips. Woodruff is highly fragrant on drying, and was traditionally used as a mattress stuffing or strewing herb.

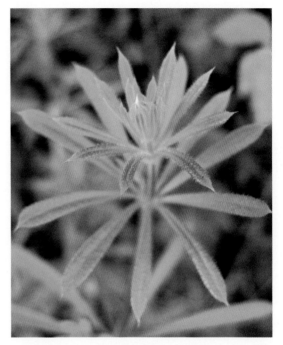

The characteristic whorls of the cleavers leaves with the spiked tips. Its hooks enable it to cleave to almost anything.

Cleavers

Where to look

Cleavers thrives in hedges and borders in most soils. It tolerates shady and sunny positions and can grow prolifically, smothering any other plants around.

When to look for it

Cleavers starts growing in February and continues right through to November. It flowers in June and sets seed in August and September.

What to harvest

The whole herb when it is fresh and green, usually before flowering.

What is it good for?

Acne vulgaris • Boils • Eczema • Psoriasis • Sore throat • Enlarged glands • Cystitis • Kidney stones

How to use it

Collect the fresh herb before it flowers when it is succulent and bright green. Make a juice of the fresh plant (this is the most potent preparation). Preserve it with alcohol or freeze it in ice-cube trays for later use. Take 1 dessertspoon, twice a day, as a spring cleansing tonic and for joint and skin disease. Make a fresh herb tincture to take for any signs of lymph congestion or swelling, such as swollen glands in tonsillitis or glandular fever. Make an infused oil of the fresh herb and apply it topically for eczema and psoriasis. Pulverize the fresh herb for use as a poultice for sores and blisters. Dry the herb and use it for infusions for its diuretic cleansing effects.

Cautions

The hooked stems can cause a skin rash.

Combines well with

Elderberry (see page 184) for viral infections with swollen glands
Dandelion root (see page 114) and plantain (see page 105) for eczema or psoriasis
Figwort (see page 53) for infected boils or acne

Forager's checklist

✳ **Perennial climbing herb**

✳ **Abundant weed**

✳ **Clinging stems, leaves and seeds**

✳ **Cooling lymphatic tonic**

✳ **Fresh herb is most effective**

✳ **Prickly hooks can cause a rash on exposed skin**

✳ **Do not confuse with woodruff**

✳ **To 1.5 m (5 ft) high**

✳ **Family: Rubiaceae**

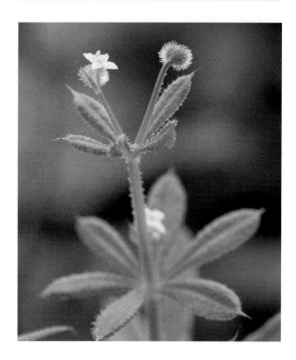

Cleaver flowers have four petals and the seeds are small, hooked balls that in some parts are called 'sweethearts'.

Glechoma hederacea

Ground ivy

ale hoof, cat's foot

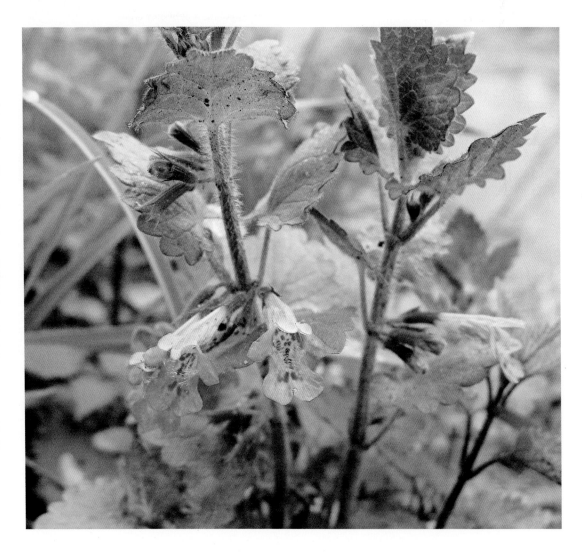

Fact and folklore

The name ale hoof derives from its ancient use as a beer flavouring by the Saxons and the leaf shape. It has a pungent, mint-like smell, due to the volatile oils it contains, and a bitter taste. The bitterness stimulates the liver, facilitating elimination of accumulated toxins. It has a reputation of being able to eliminate lead from the body if exposure to it from old water pipes has been a problem. Its bitterness is effective for gently stimulating the digestion and will improve a poor appetite, especially if it is associated with mucous congestion and being 'full of cold'.

The aromatic element works as an antiseptic decongestant that can help to unblock congested nasal passages and increase expectoration of mucus from the lungs. Its tannin content means it is also a mucous membrane astringent and will tone up inflamed membranes that are producing lots of secretions. By improving their tone, it makes them less susceptible to irritation to allergens. It is particularly useful in hayfever, for sinusitis and for children with runny noses and poor appetite. It may be used as an eyebath for itching eye symptoms of hayfever and for conjunctivitis and styes. The volatile oils are also diuretic and can be taken to increase flow of urine in bladder infections and to help flush out kidney stones.

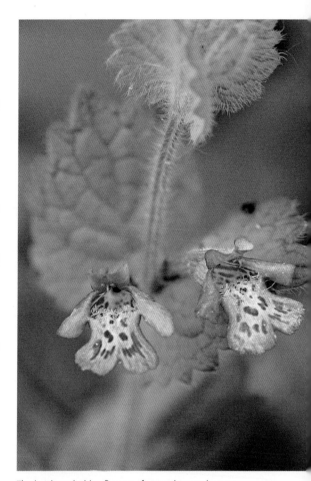

The bright violet-blue flowers of ground ivy make it an attractive plant that provides dense ground cover in the spring.

What to look for

Ground ivy is a perennial plant that grows up to 20 cm (8 in) high and 60 cm (24 in) wide. The roots send out long, trailing, unbranched, square stems. It has dark green leaves that are characteristically hairy, kidney-shaped and with round, toothed edges. The leaves sit opposite each other on the stems. The purple flowers are three-lobed above and two-lobed below. They have deeper purple and white spots on the lower part leading to the stamen and anther deep inside the flower. The whole plant is aromatic.

Can be mistaken for

Ground ivy has a characteristic pungent, mint-like scent that makes it difficult to confuse with any other plant.

Where to look

The plant grows in waste ground, wood margins and hedge banks.

When to look for it

Ground ivy grows and flowers from April to November.

What to harvest

The whole flowering plant.

What is it good for?

Bruises • Conjunctivitis • Catarrh • Colds • Coughs • Earache • Hayfever • Sinusitis • Indigestion • Cystitis • Kidney stones

How to use it

Gather the fresh herb while in flower and make a tincture. Take a teaspoon of this before meals to improve appetite and digestion, and for blood cleansing and mucous membrane tonic effects. Harvest the fresh herb and use fresh or dry for infusions to drink and for eyedrops or eyewashes. Use a warm infusion with a pinch of salt added as a nasal douche for sinusitis every four hours to flush out bacteria. Take an infusion of the fresh or dried herb to encourage expectoration of thick phlegm in chesty coughs, and for urinary problems. Allow the infusion to cool and drink frequently for acute conditions of the urinary tract, like cystitis. Make a poultice of the fresh herb by bruising it well, and place it over bruises to speed healing, repeating two or three times a day.

Cautions

Do not use as an independent treatment for lead toxicity without consulting a medical practitioner.

Forager's checklist

* **Common, creeping perennial plant**
* **Widely distributed**
* **Unusual scent when crushed**
* **Long flowering period**
* **Decongestant**
* **20 cm (8 in) high and 60 cm (24 in) wide**
* **Family: Labiatae**

Combines well with

Elderflower (see page 184), eyebright (see page 96) and elecampane (see page 140) for catarrh
Couch grass (see page 90) and yarrow (see page 84) for urinary problems
Eyebright (see page 96) for a soothing eyewash

Try it in ground ivy nasal douche

Sinuses are a breeding ground for bacteria, but by directly rinsing out the nasal cavities, infective organisms are flushed away. The tonic properties of herbs can then have a direct effect on the mucous membranes, rather than having to be absorbed by the digestive tract and carried there by the blood. Use a cup of warm infusion of 5 g (1 teaspoon) ground ivy herb with 5–10 g (1–2 teaspoons) salt. Block one nostril and sniff the infusion into the other nostril until it runs down the back of the throat. Then spit it out of the mouth. Repeat until the nostril is clear, then repeat on the other nostril. Do this every few hours to gain relief from sinusitis and colds and to aid recovery.

Ground ivy

Humulus lupulus

Hop
golden hop

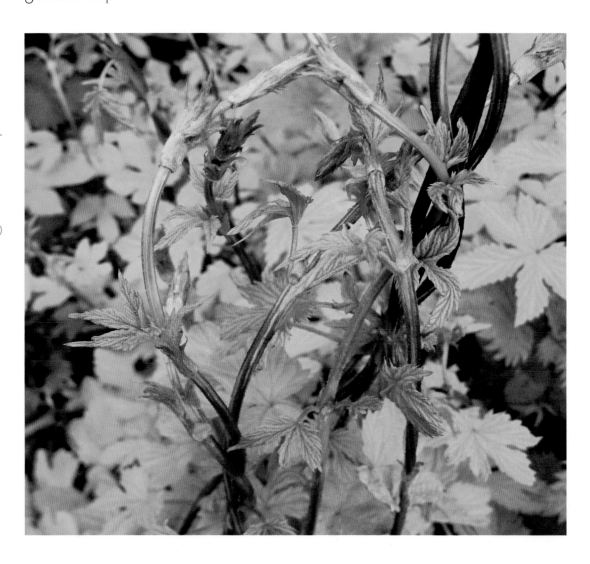

Fact and folklore

The name hop comes from the Anglo Saxon *hoppen*, meaning 'to climb'. The young, sprouting stems, which resemble wild asparagus, were cooked and eaten in the spring, and were gathered and sold in bunches. Hops are used for flavouring beer, and can be seen growing in the famous hop fields of Kent in southern England. They are considered to reduce sexual desire, and have hormonal actions that can be used in menopause for low oestrogen levels. Hops have a sedative effect on the nervous system. The relaxing action works on colic pains and is also useful for gallbladder spasm. Hops are also bitter and encourage efficient liver function and also an improved digestive function.

What to look for

The hop is a perennial climbing plant. The stems arise in a mass of angular, hooked shoots that climb up any adjacent plant or structure to 2–6 m (6–20 ft) high. The pale green, slightly rough leaves are three-lobed and have finely toothed edges. The flowers are male or female and found on separate plants – it is the female flower that is used medicinally (the male flower is tiny). The female flower is cone-like and scented, and leaves the fingers gritty and sticky after picking.

Can be mistaken for

White bryony (*Bryonia dioica*) has a similar hedge-climbing habit and similar three-lobed leaves. It is bright green, smooth to the touch and has tendrils that wrap themselves tightly around anchor points to help it climb. The flowers are small and white, and it bear strings of bright red berries in the autumn. It is poisonous.

Hop

Where to look

Hops grow in hedgerows and up any poles within them. They are found throughout Europe – introduced in Scotland and rare in Ireland.

When to look for it

From midsummer the plant will have grown high enough to emerge from the hedge top. It flowers from late August to mid-September.

What to harvest

The cone-like flowers.

What is it good for?

Anxiety and stress • Insomnia • Colic • Diverticular disease • Gallstones • Irritable bowel syndrome (IBS) • Menopause

How to use it

Gather the flowers and dry them to make a fragrant tincture. The tincture needs to be made with 60 per cent alcohol to extract the resins. The flowers may also be dried and used for a bitter infusion. Take a cool infusion before bed to aid sleep that is disturbed by hot flushes. Make a hop pillow (see page 180).

Cautions

Do not use in depression.

Combines well with

Valerian (see page 79) for insomnia
Chamomile (see page 102) and mint (see page 198) for irritable bowel syndrome (IBS)
Cramp bark (see page 187) and fumitory (see page 99) or dandelion root (see page 114) for gallstones

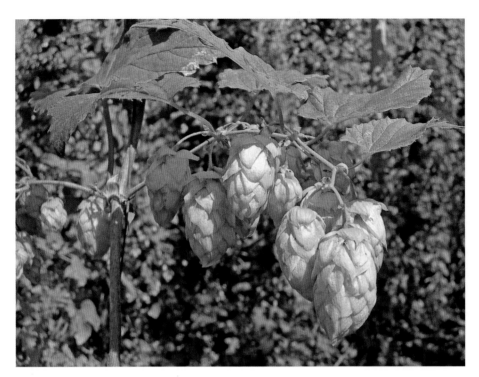

The female hop flowers grow on a separate plant to the male hop flowers, which are much smaller.

Try it in a hop pillow

You will need a 30 cm (12 in) square of cotton fabric, two 28 cm (11 in) squares of cotton wadding and 25 g (1 oz) freshly dried hops. Sew together three sides of the fabric with the right side facing inward, and then turn it the right side out. Insert the two squares of wadding. Put the hops into the pillow between the layers of wadding, spreading them evenly throughout. Turn the edges in on the open side and sew the pillow shut. To stop the hops gathering in one area, sew across the pillow eight times at 7.5 cm (3 in) intervals, quilting it into a grid. Place on the pillow of someone in need of a good night's sleep, giving it a squeeze to release the scent.

Forager's checklist

* **Perennial hedgerow climber**
* **Widely distributed**
* **Depressant action on nerves**
* **Use cone-like female flowers**
* **Harvest flowers in early autumn**
* **2–6 m (6–20 ft) high**
* **Family: Cannabaceae**

Lamium album

White deadnettle

archangel

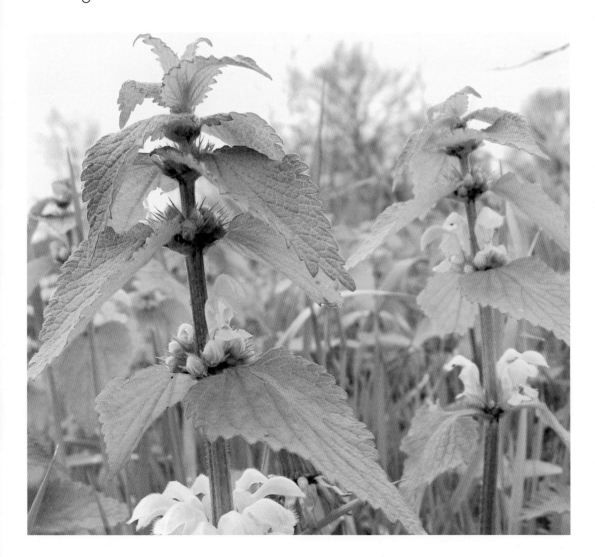

Fact and folklore

Although the deadnettle resembles the stinging nettle (see page 155), it belongs to a different plant family. It is referred to as 'dead' because its fine hairs do not sting. Its close resemblance to the stinging nettle, and the fact that it often grows among stinging nettles, is a clever adaptation by which it gives itself some protection from grazing animals and leaf-eating insects. Bees love it as it contains large quantities of nectar. If you pluck the flower from its calyx and gently suck the base, the nectar will taste sweet on your tongue.

The whole herb is rich in tannins and its astringent effects are used generally for bleeding conditions. There is not much modern research into the use of deadnettle, but traditionally it was used in heavy and prolonged menstrual bleeding and for balancing the hormones. This action continues to be exploited by current herbalists. It is a gentle herb and needs at least three menstrual cycles to have an effect. It is also used for uninfected vaginal discharge, where its tannins will tone up the mucous membranes of the vaginal walls, and may also be used for uninfected diarrhoea, to tone the bowel walls.

What to look for

White deadnettle has a widely spreading root system that sends up many new shoots distant from the parent plant, and grows 15–25 cm (6–10 in) high. The stems are square and hollow, and they bear heart-shaped leaves with fine soft hairs and serrated edges. The small flowers form in whorls on the stem and are white and trumpet-shaped, with small black spots and hairs inside that lead pollinators to the nectar at the base. The green spiked calyx remains after the petals have dropped and holds the seeds inside in tight pods until ripe.

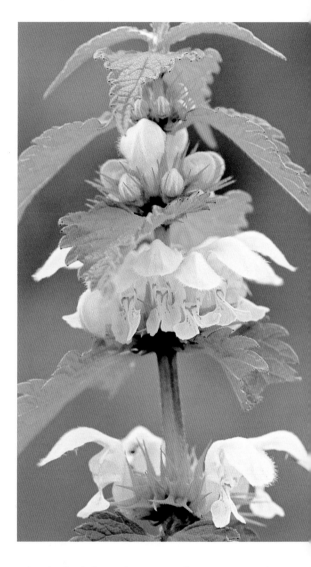

White deadnettle flowers have a taste of sweet nectar – pick them out and gently suck the base for a sweet treat.

Can be mistaken for

Before it flowers, it looks like the stinging nettle (see page 155) and other deadnettles, such as the red or purple deadnettle (*Lamium purpureum*), which has more heart-shaped leaves.

Where to look

White deadnettle is found growing in most soils in hedgerows, meadows, waste ground and gardens.

When to look for it

The plant can be found growing all year round and flowers from March to December.

What to harvest

The whole flowering plant.

What is it good for?

Diarrhoea • Heavy periods

How to use it

Gather the fresh herb when in flower and infuse it for internal use for menstrual irregularities with heavy or excessive bleeding. Use the cooled infusion as a mouthwash or vaginal douche for excessive simple discharges. The herb maintains its properties on drying and may be stored for use in dry herb infusions. Alternatively, make a fresh herb tincture for easy regular use and for combination with other herbs.

Cautions

Do not take for infected conditions without treating the infection too. For prolonged or unexplained vaginal bleeding or changed bowel habits, always consult your doctor or a medical herbalist.

Forager's checklist

* ❋ **Perennial weed**
* ❋ **Widely distributed**
* ❋ **Frequently growing all year**
* ❋ **Long flowering period**
* ❋ **No sting**
* ❋ **Use whole plant**
* ❋ **Astringent tonic**
* ❋ **15–25 cm (6–10 in) high**
* ❋ **Family: Labiatae**

Combines well with

Shepherd's purse (see page 131) and nettle (see page 155) for excessive menstrual bleeding

Try it in tea for heavy menstrual bleeding

This is a pleasant-tasting infusion of herbs that are rich in blood vessel-toning tannins that have an affinity for the female reproductive system, especially the uterus. It is important to have an understanding of why heavy menstrual bleeding is occurring and undertake to address that with appropriate measures. Combine equal parts of the following dried herbs: white deadnettle; shepherd's purse; nettle and rose petals. Make an infusion of 25 g (1 oz) to 600 ml (1 pint) boiling water and drink 1 cupful three times a day for at least two menstrual cycles.

White deadnettle

Sambucus nigra

Elder

black elder, Judas tree, witches' tree

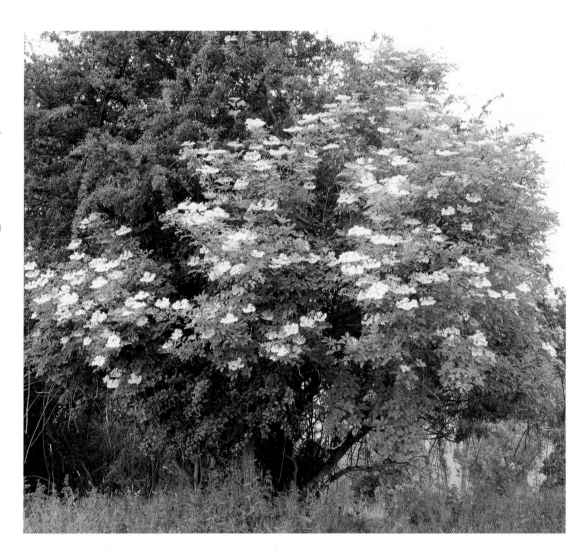

Fact and folklore

Elder has always been valued for its medicinal properties, and workers laying hedges often would not cut it because it was so valued for medicine. Both the flowers and berries make a delicious tonic wine. It is used for colds, chills, fevers, viral infections and as a source of vitamin C. The berries have recently been shown to have antiviral properties and to inhibit the flu virus. The flowers are tonic for the mucous membranes of the nose and sinuses, and are useful for colds, sinusitis and hayfever. They also induce sweating in fevers. The flowers are emollient and moisturizing for the skin.

What to look for

Elder is a large shrub, up to 6 m (20 ft) tall, with oval, pointed, finely serrated leaves. The bark on the old wood feels slightly spongy. It bears flat-topped bunches of frothy, tiny, creamy-white, five-petalled flowers – their stamens are thick with pollen and strongly scented. The flowers develop into bunches of tiny, shiny berries that are initially green and turn first red then purple-black. The flowers have an unusual heavy scent that grows stronger while drying but becomes pleasant when they are dry.

Can be mistaken for

Cramp bark (see page 187) has a similar flowering habit.

Where to look

Elder grows almost anywhere and can be found in hedgerows, field boundaries, woods and waste ground.

When to look for it

The shrub grows from April to October. It flowers in May and the berries ripen at the end of August.

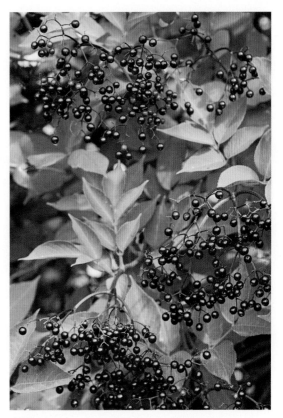

Elderberries are an abundant source of Vitamin C and extracts have been shown to have antiviral properties.

Elder

What to harvest

The flowers in spring when white and heavy with pollen. The berries in September when they are ripe.

What is it good for?

Conjunctivitis • Eczema • Psoriasis • Catarrh • Colds • Flu • Hayfever • Sinusitis • Sore throat • Chickenpox and shingles • Allergies • Fever • Infection • Constipation • Cystitis

How to use it

Harvest the flowers when they are creamy-white and heavy with pollen, snipping them off the stems, and dry them for use as infusions. The cold infusion can be used as a soothing eyewash for irritated, infected or itching eyes, or added to baths for dry skin conditions. Make fresh elderflower tincture and syrup. The syrup can be diluted with cold water and makes a pleasant drink. Make an infused oil of the flowers and use as a moisturizing skin oil or ointment for dry eczema and psoriasis.

Harvest the berries when they turn purple and are rich and shiny. Dry them for use in decoctions, or make elderberry syrup for a delicious hot drink in the winter. Make fresh elderberry tincture that can be combined 50:50 with the syrup to make elderberry compound; take 1 teaspoon every hour at the first sign of sore throat or a cold. Eat them whole, raw or cooked for a laxative effect.

Cautions

Elderberries may be laxative if taken raw in large quantities.

Combines well with

Mint (see page 198) and yarrow (see page 84) for colds, flu and fever
Ground ivy (see page 175) and nettle (see page 155) for hayfever

Try it in elderberry syrup

Gather the elderberries when they are fully ripe on a dry day. Strip them from their stems with a fork. Put into a pan with a small amount of water, enough to cover the bottom of the pan and prevent the berries from burning. Bring them up to the boil. Turn the heat down and simmer them until they give up their juice, which will take about 25 minutes. Strain them and press through a muslin or fine-meshed sieve. Measure the volume of liquid and add 375 g (12 oz) sugar for each 600 ml (1 pint) of liquid. Put back in the pan with 10 cloves and 2.5 cm (1 in) fresh ginger or half a teaspoon dried powdered ginger for each 600 ml (1 pint). Put back on the heat and stir until all the sugar has dissolved. Bring up to the boil for five minutes. Then strain into sterilized bottles. Store in the refrigerator when opened. It will keep for up to a year but discard before if it develops mould. Dilute to taste with hot or cold water or make elderberry compound, see above.

Forager's checklist

- **Large deciduous shrub**
- **Frothy bunches of creamy-white flowers**
- **Bunches of purple-black berries**
- **Berries stain clothing and fingers**
- **Flowers are a mucous membrane tonic**
- **Berries are antiviral**
- **6 m (20 ft) tall**
- **Family: Caprifoliaceae**

Viburnum opulus

Cramp bark

guelder rose, red elder

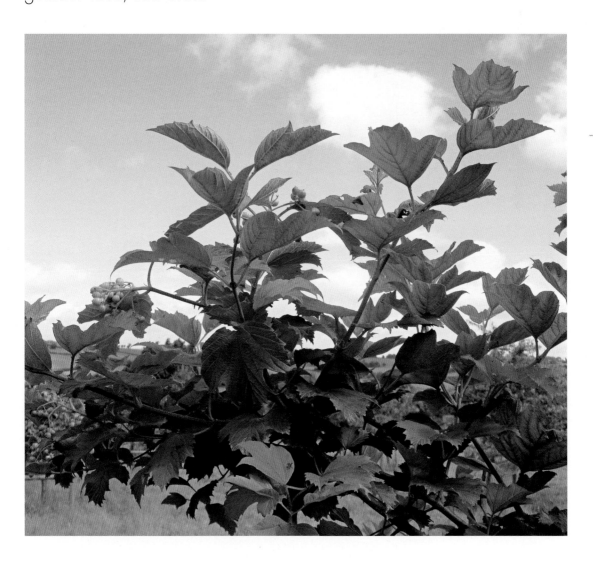

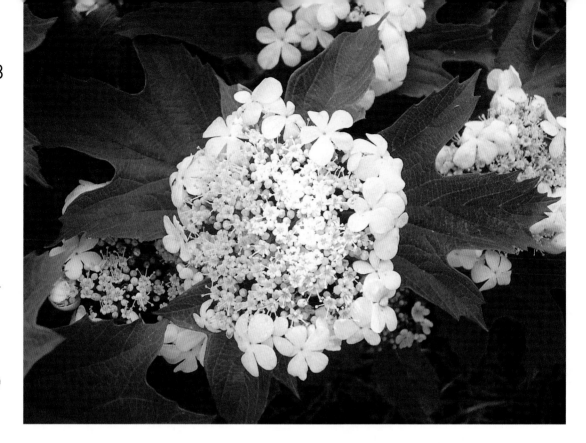

Fact and folklore

The name guelder rose comes from the fact that this plant originated in Gueldersland, a Dutch province, where it was first cultivated. It belongs to the same family as elder and they do resemble each other, which is why it is also known as red elder. It is further known as cramp bark because the bark has antispasmodic properties and is used for relaxing tension and spasm of hollow organs and muscles. It can be used for period pains and the pain from stones in renal and biliary colic. It relaxes the smooth muscles of the blood vessels, so is used for high blood pressure. It can be taken for spasmodic colicky pains in the bowels and the symptoms of irritable bowel

The cramp bark flower is differentiated from elderflowers by the large, showy, sterile flowers on the edge of the blooms.

syndrome. When cramp bark is applied topically to the skin, it will relax spasms and cramps of skeletal muscles.

What to look for

Viburnum is a tall shrub, up to 5 m (16 ft) in height, with smooth, grey bark and light green, three-lobed, maple-like leaves. It produces large, flat-topped flower clusters with large, white, sterile flowers around the edge and smaller, pollen-bearing flowers in the centre. Bunches of large, red berries follow the flowers.

Can be mistaken for

Elder (see page 184) has a similar growing habit and is found in the same places, but elder has bipinnate leaves (see page 20) and its flower clusters are made entirely of tiny, creamy-white flowers.

Where to look

It is a common hedgerow plant.

When to look for it

Cramp bark grows from May to October. Harvest the bark in spring just as the leaves start to unfurl.

What to harvest

The bark. Do not strip it from growing branches, but from prunings.

What is it good for?

Backache • Cramp • Restless leg syndrome • Chilblains • High blood pressure • Headache • Colic • Diverticular disease • Gallstones • Irritable bowel syndrome (IBS) • Kidney stones • Painful periods

How to use it

Dry the bark for use in decoctions to relieve the pain from kidney stones, gallstones and bowel spasm. Or make a tincture of the fresh bark to use for period pains, to relax the uterus. Use it in combination with other herbs for high blood pressure, especially if tension and anxiety are contributing factors. For muscle cramps or tension, make a rubbing liniment with it and massage into the affected muscle.

Cautions

If treating high blood pressure, it is advisable to do so with the assistance of a registered medical herbalist and your doctor. Be aware of the risks of kidney stone or gallstone impaction.

Combines well with

Fumitory (see page 99) and hop (see page 178) for gallstones
Lime (see page 56) and hawthorn (see page 166) for high blood pressure
Dandelion leaf (see page 114) for kidney stones

Try it in cramp bark liniment

Mix 50 ml (2 fl oz) chamomile-infused oil, 20 ml (^{3}/$_4$ fl oz) cramp bark tincture and 20 ml (^{3}/$_4$ fl oz) valerian tincture in a 100 ml (3^1/$_2$ fl oz) glass bottle and shake well. Massage well into the affected area. This will keep for up to a year.

Forager's checklist

* **Deciduous shrub**
* **Widely distributed**
* **Bright red berries**
* **Smooth muscle relaxant**
* **Harvest bark in spring**
* **Take bark from prunings**
* **5 m (16 ft) tall**
* **Family: Caprifoliaceae**

Cramp bark

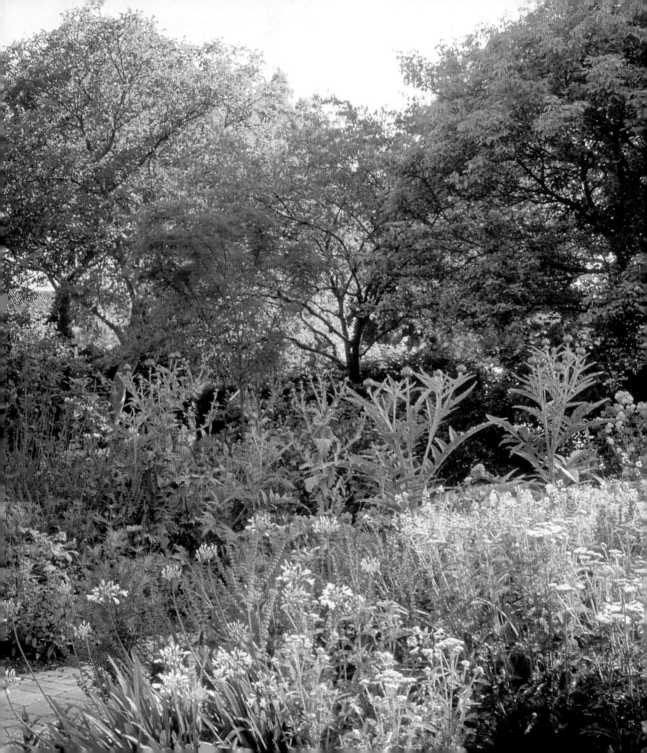

GARDEN VISITORS

Many cottage gardens still contain medicinal plants that were
specially cultivated for their properties in years gone by, remedies
remembered and used by country folk who relied on them for
healing simple ailments. Other healing plants may be introduced
by the gardener or find their own way to the garden. Take time
to discover and treasure the special qualities of the healing plants
that grow in every garden, from the grandest estate to the
smallest yard.

Bellis perennis

Daisy

bruisewort

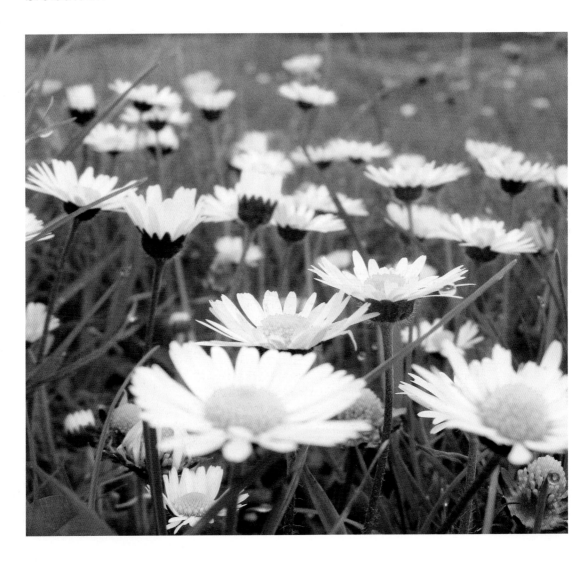

Fact and folklore

Some say that *Bellis perennis* means 'always beautiful', but it is also possible that *Bellis* derives from the Latin *bellum* meaning 'war', as it was traditionally used on battlefields to staunch the flow of blood from wounds. It is one of the first flowers known by children for making daisy chains and for playing 'he loves me, he loves me not', and in Scotland it is known as 'bairnwort' because children love to play with it. The common name comes from 'day's eye', as the flowers open and close with sunrise and sunset.

In the Doctrine of Signatures, it resembles an eye and has been traditionally used as an eyewash for eye conditions and black eyes. It has similar uses to the better-known arnica, but grows prolifically and is more readily available. Daisy has astringent properties and is useful as a topical application for bruises. It may also be applied for dilated blood vessels in the red noses and cheeks of acne rosacea and to relieve irritation from haemorrhoids (piles). Use it as a wash for weeping skin problems such as varicose eczema. It has diuretic properties and can be taken internally to flush toxins from the system in skin and joint disease.

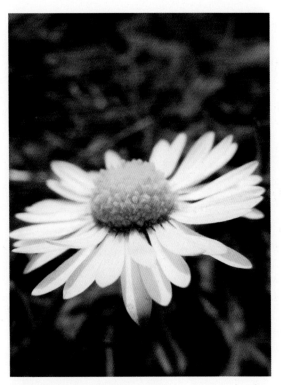

The name daisy comes from 'day's eye' as it opens when the sun rises and closes when the sun sets.

Daisy

What to look for

Daisy is a low-growing perennial, 7.5 cm (3 in) tall and 15 cm (6 in) wide. It arises from a shallow root system with spoon-shaped leaves forming a basal rosette. It grows many round stalks with a single flower at the top. The flowers have many long, white petals around the edge and the centre is bright yellow.

Can be mistaken for

Ox-eye daisy (*Leucanthemum vulgare*) is a tall, often cultivated, showy daisy with large flowers that has similar medicinal properties.

Where to look

Very common in short grass everywhere including lawns, footpaths, verges and grazed meadows.

When to look for it

The daisy grows all year round; it may also flower during mild winters.

What to harvest

The whole plant, preferably in flower. The daisy flowers may be used on their own for use in a fresh herb poultice.

Garden visitors

What is it good for?
Acne rosacea • Bruises • Arthritis • Gout • Sprains and strains • Haemorrhoids (piles)

How to use it
Daisies are virtually always available as a fresh herb. Pick the whole plant, pulverize it slightly and use as a poultice on bumps and bruises. Make an infused oil of the fresh plant for use in salves and ointments. Make an infusion of the fresh herb for use as a compress or enema for piles. Use a fresh infusion daily as a lotion for redness of the nose and face and for varicose eczema. Make a fresh herb tincture for use internally for gout and arthritis and chronic skin disease.

Cautions
Do not take internally if digestive bleeding or irritation is a problem. It is advised to take this herb with the supervision of a medical herbalist.

Forager's checklist
❋ **Perennial herb**
❋ **Widely distributed**
❋ **Good for bruising**
❋ **Harvest all year**
❋ **Use the whole plant**
❋ **7.5 cm (3 in) tall and 15 cm (6 in) wide**
❋ **Family: Compositae**

Combines well with
Horse chestnut (see page 38) for haemorrhoids (piles)
Yarrow (see page 84) as a wash for varicose eczema

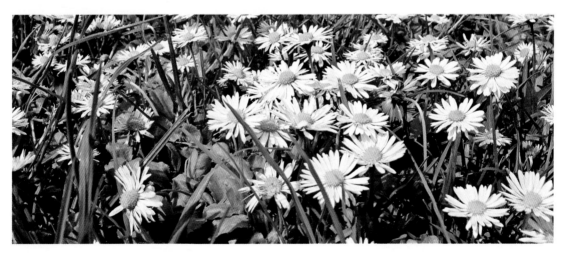

A joyful addition to any lawn, daisies flower all year round providing fresh medicine whenever it is needed.

Carduus marianum (syn. Silybum marianum)

Milk thistle

marian thistle

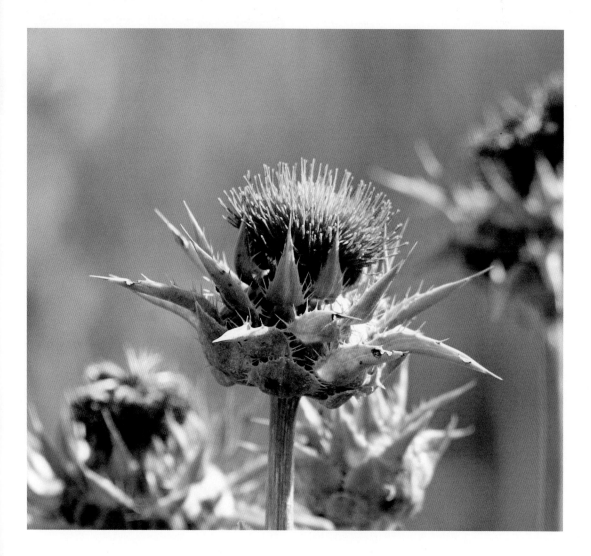

Garden visitors

Fact and folklore

Milk thistle has long been used for liver problems, and modern science has now shown that it is a powerful liver remedy. It protects the cells of the liver from damage from all kinds of toxins and can help the cells regenerate. It is used in the treatment of all degenerative liver diseases, including hepatitis and cirrhosis caused by over-consumption of alcohol. It may be used prior to drinking alcohol to protect against potential damage, and afterwards to help the liver eliminate alcohol from the system.

Skin conditions such as eczema, acne and psoriasis often partly arise from poor liver function, making milk thistle a useful herb to take. The liver also plays a part in formation of lipo proteins from cholesterol so supporting its function in the treatment of cholesterol problems is of value. If there has been any exposure to environmental toxins, milk thistle is essential to support the liver function. It has a traditional use to increase breast milk.

What to look for

Milk thistle is a biennial plant, 60–120 cm (2–4 ft) high and 30 cm (1 ft) wide, producing a basal rosette of deeply cut, wavy leaves in the first year. Each lobe of the leaf is tipped with a sharp point, and the veins of the leaf are pure white. In the second year, the flower grows on top of a long stem. The calyx forms a large, scaled, spiked, green, globe-shaped base with many purple florets emerging from the top. The pale brown or buff seeds are small and oval.

Can be mistaken for

Other members of the thistle family have similar leaves and flowers but without the clear white veins on the leaves.

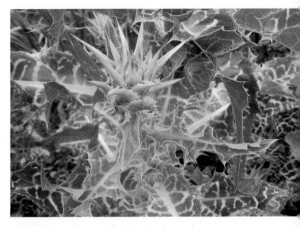

Milk thistle can be identified by the clear, white veins running through its wavy, pointed leaves.

Where to look

Milk thistle grows on rough and waste ground as a garden escapee. It is rare in Scotland, but is easily cultivated in gardens.

When to look for it

In the first year, it produces a basal rosette of leaves. In the second year, it flowers in July.

What to harvest

The seeds.

What is it good for?

Acne rosacea • Acne vulgaris • Psoriasis • Gout • Atherosclerosis • High cholesterol • Allergies • Bloating • Gallstones • Hangover • Indigestion • Premenstrual tension (PMT)

How to use it

Harvest the seeds and make into a fresh herb tincture for use as a liver protector before and after alcohol consumption. Take the tincture regularly as a part of treatment for skin disease or for conditions requiring liver support. If it is being used for liver disease, to avoid alcohol from the tincture, grind the seeds and sprinkle 1 teaspoon on food 2–3 times a day, or mix in a glass of water and drink. The finely ground seed may also be put into capsules – take 2 capsules twice a day.

Cautions
Prescribed medications may potentially be affected by taking milk thistle. Consult a medical herbalist.

Combines well with
Nettle (see page 155) to increase the production of breast milk

Try it in milk thistle powder
If milk thistle is going to be ground and used sprinkled on food, it is important to know that ground herbs lose their potency faster than whole herbs; after three months their medicinal qualities are substantially reduced. Grind enough for a few weeks at a time and store it in a glass jar in a cool, dark place. Milk thistle has a tough outer coat that is difficult to grind manually in a pestle and mortar. Grind either in an electric coffee bean grinder or in the blender jug on a food processor. Milk thistle seed is mildly bitter to taste, but it combines very well with ground pumpkin and sunflower seeds – this mix makes it a more palatable, highly nutritious addition to cereal, yogurt or stewed fruit. It may also be stirred into water and drunk down. Use 1 teaspoon of powder twice a day to assist liver function during times of stress, for hormone excess, high cholesterol levels, as a liver cell protector prior to alcohol consumption, for sluggish digestion and feelings of toxicity following over-indulgence.

Forager's checklist
* **Self-seeding biennial**
* **Widely distributed**
* **White-veined, prickly leaves**
* **Attractive large, purple-flowering thistle heads**
* **Liver protector**
* **Supports liver cell regeneration**
* **Use the seeds**
* **Harvest after flowering**
* **60–120 cm (2–4 ft) high and 30 cm (1 ft) wide**
* **Family: Compositae**

Milk thistle

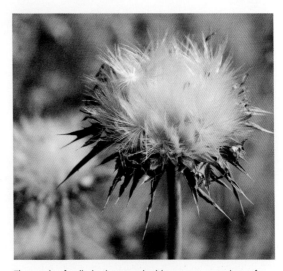

The seeds of milk thistle are valuable protective medicine for the liver, which can struggle with excessive modern lifestyles.

Mentha spp.

Mint

peppermint, horsemint, spearmint, watermint

Garden visitors

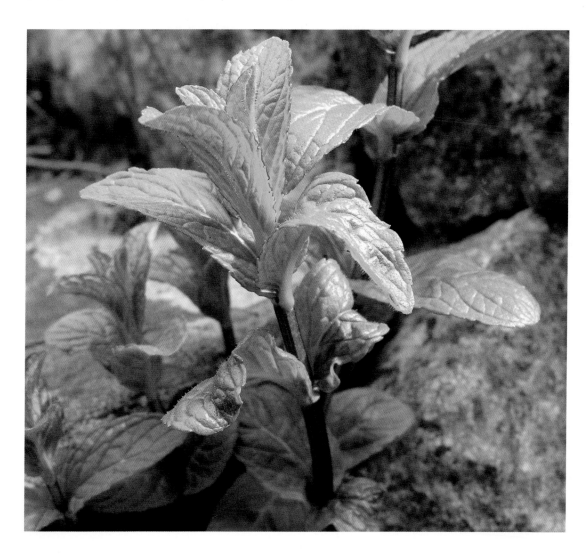

Fact and folklore

Peppermint and spearmint were introduced to Britain by the Romans, who cultivated them for their medicinal and culinary virtues. They have become naturalized and may often be found growing in the wild. Mint is used as a digestive antispasmodic for discomfort from wind, bloating and colic. It may also alleviate nausea and can sometimes halt the onset of migraine or headache. Mint is a good decongestant and is used for catarrh and to relieve the symptoms of colds and sinusitis. Externally, the commercially bought essential oil is analgesic and is used to freeze out pain from muscle sprains, strains and tension. It will also relieve itching skin.

What to look for

The fresh, cleansing scent is common to all the mints, although may vary slightly from plant to plant. The basic structure is also the same. Peppermint (*Mentha* x *piperita*) is described in detail here. It grows 40–60 cm (16–24 in) high and 60 cm (24 in) wide from a spreading root system that sends up new shoots, and is locally invasive. The stems are square with elongated, finely serrated leaves. The pale purple flowers form as tight whorls around the stem with small leaves emerging at their bases; the flower whorls diminish in size further up the stem.

Can be mistaken for

Horsemint (*Mentha longifolia*) is like a hairy version of spearmint, and watermint (*M. aquatica*) is possibly indigenous to Europe. There are many crosses between species, but the medicinal properties are similar, with some varieties being milder than others. Corn mint (*M. arvensis*) and round-leaved mint (*M. suaveolens*) have similar properties, as does pennyroyal

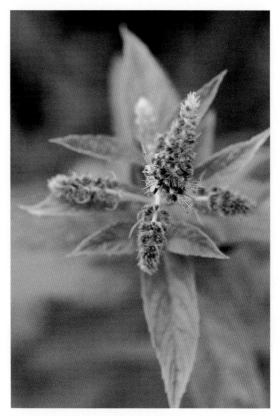

The sharp scent of mint clears congested nasal passages and infused in a tea stimulates the digestion.

(*M. pulegium*), but avoid the latter in pregnancy (see 'Cautions' on page 200).

Where to look

Mint is often found in cottage gardens, on waste ground and near water.

When to look for it

Mint is a perennial herb that grows from March to October. It flowers from June to October.

Mint

Garden visitors

What to harvest
The leaves.

What is it good for?
Catarrh • Colds • Flu • Sinusitis • Headache •
Migraine • Fever • Bloating • Colic • Diarrhoea •
Diverticular disease • Flatulence • Irritable bowel
syndrome (IBS) • Nausea

How to use it
Gather the leaves and use fresh or dried as an infusion
to drink on a regular basis for irritable bowel or
flatulence. A strong infusion may halt a headache or
migraine. Make a fresh herb tincture to preserve all its
properties, particularly the volatile oils, some of which
are lost on drying. Use the tincture diluted or a cooled
infusion as a wash for itching, or combine the tincture
into a base cream for muscular pain – however, the
essential oil is most effective for this.

Cautions
The antispasmodic effect may aggravate indigestion
and heartburn. Do not use pennyroyal (*M. pulegium*)
during pregnancy as it is a strong uterine stimulant.

Combines well with
Chamomile (see page 102) and hop (see page 178) for
irritable bowel syndrome (IBS) and colic
Yarrow (see page 84) and elderflower (see page 184)
for colds, fevers and flu
Wood betony (see page 111) for headache

Try it in Moroccan mint tea
This tea is an excellent digestive and pick-me-up for
after meals that will reduce digestive fermentation
and disperse wind. It is traditionally served in Morocco

Forager's checklist
❋ **Perennial herb**
❋ **Often escaped from cultivation**
❋ **Many varieties and cross-breeds**
❋ **Prolific growth**
❋ **Regenerates quickly from harvesting**
❋ **New plants from smallest root cutting**
❋ **Familiar fresh scent**
❋ **Digestive carminative**
❋ **May halt onset of headaches**
❋ **Use fresh or dried**
❋ **Harvest the leaves**
❋ **40–60 cm (16–24 in) high and 60 cm (24 in) wide**
❋ **Family: Labiatae**

following meals. The green tea may be omitted to
avoid caffeine. It may also be drunk between meals as
a digestive carminative to settle an upset digestive
tract. Also try it at the first sign of a migraine to allay
nausea; it may also prevent the migraine from
developing fully. For each person, use 1 teaspoon
green tea (or gunpowder tea which is green tea rolled
into balls), 12 mint leaves and 3–5 teaspoons sugar to
taste. Put the green tea, mint leaves and sugar into a
pot and pour over boiling water. Leave to infuse for
five minutes. Serve the tea in a tall glass with a few
extra mint leaves packed in the bottom.

Tanacetum parthenium

Feverfew

featherfew

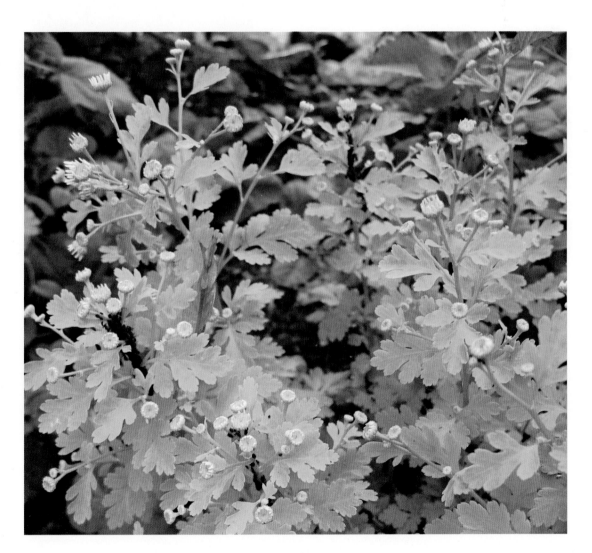

Fact and folklore

The name feverfew comes from the word 'febrifuge', as it was traditionally used to dispel fever. It was commonly used as a herb for hysteria and nervousness and will bring on delayed menstruation. It was also used topically as a poultice to reduce the pain and swelling of insect bites and stings. Modern research has demonstrated that it has abilities to moderate the effects of histamine, inflammatory prostaglandin substances and can reduce blood clotting. The properties are similar to those of aspirin, but it is thought to work via different mechanisms.

Feverfew is most commonly known for the treatment of migraines, reducing the tension and inflammation that causes the typical thumping, pressure pain. It is used as a prophylactic for migraines and can also be taken at the onset. It is rich in niacin, which dilates the blood vessels; this may explain its effects in the treatment of migraines, as they are known to be caused by tension and then engorgement of the blood vessels in the brain. Feverfew also has gentle sedative effects, aiding relaxation and easing pain. Its anti-inflammatory properties also make it useful for spasmodic, cramping menstrual pains and for swollen, painful joints. Its bitter properties have a stimulant effect on the liver and are good for the digestion and improving appetite.

What to look for

This attractive herb grows 30–50 cm (12–20 in) tall and wide, and has dense, lacy, fern-like foliage. The whole plant has a citrusy, pungent scent. Pale green, deeply cut leaves grow alternately on a round stem. Tall, branching stems bear many flat, daisy-like flowers with large, white petals around the edge and many yellow, densely packed florets in the centre.

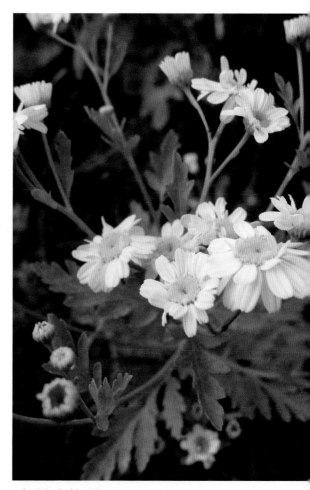

A fresh leaf of feverfew eaten everyday is said to ward off migraines; however, it may irritate sensitive mouths.

Can be mistaken for

German chamomile (*Matricaria recutita*; see page 102) has leaves that are finely and deeply cut and the flowers are conical rather than flat. The scent of chamomile is more delicate and sweeter than that of feverfew.

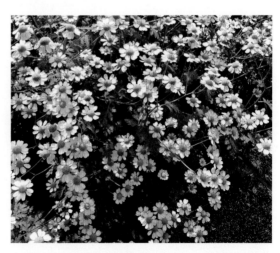

Where to look

Feverfew is common on waste ground and arable field margins. It is also often found in cottage gardens, as it was much cultivated for its medicinal properties.

When to look for it

Feverfew grows from April to November and flowers from July to September.

What to harvest

The whole plant just before it flowers.

What is it good for?

Arthritis • Migraine • Painful periods

How to use it

Make a fresh herb tincture, as feverfew loses most of its properties on drying. For period pains, take a standard dose of this tincture a few days before menstruation. Take it as a standard dose at the first sign of a migraine. Take a fresh leaf every day as a prophylactic against migraines.

Cautions

Some people are sensitive to this herb and experience mouth blisters from eating it raw. Do not use during pregnancy.

Combines well with

Wood betony (see page 111) for migraine and headaches
Cramp bark (see page 187) for period pains

Try it in a feverfew sandwich

Put a fresh leaf in a sandwich every day as a treatment for migraines; the bread should protect the inside of

Forager's checklist

* **Perennial herb**
* **Widely distributed**
* **Flat, daisy-like flowers**
* **Good for migraines**
* **Use whole herb**
* **Harvest before flowering**
* **30–50 cm (12–20 in) tall and wide**
* **Family: Compositae**

Feverfew

the mouth against its potentially caustic effects. Alternatively, roll the leaf up, squash it into a small ball of bread and swallow.

The flowers of feverfew bloom for a long time; the fresh plant is more effective than when it is dried.

Thymus serpyllum

Wild thyme

mother of thyme

Garden visitors

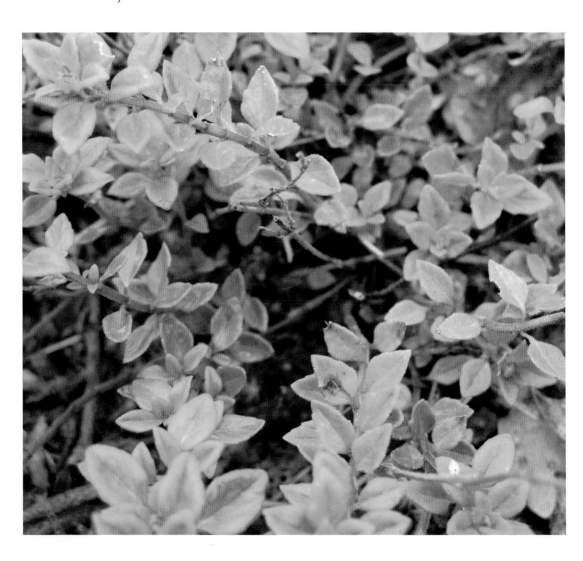

Fact and folklore

Wild thyme is much smaller than common garden thyme (*Thymus vulgaris*) and the name *serpyllum* comes from Greek, meaning 'to creep'. Bees love thyme blossom and its healing properties are passed on in their honey; thyme honey is a powerful anti-infective wound agent. Thyme is also an excellent digestive remedy, easing intestinal spasm and dispersing wind, and its strong flavour makes it a popular culinary herb.

Thyme contains volatile oils that open the airways and relieve wheezing, loosens thick mucus and encourages expectoration, which is good for most respiratory problems. Thyme has potent antiseptic properties, and can be taken as a mouthwash or gargle for a sore throat, oral thrush and inflamed or infected gums. It is also antifungal and is a good treatment for thrush and other fungal infections such as athlete's foot.

What to look for

Wild thyme is a small, creeping plant, 10–15 cm (4–6 in) high and 30 cm (12 in) wide, that can spread over large areas. The leaves are minute, and the small flowers are pinky-purple and trumpet-shaped, splitting at the wide end into four lobes.

Can be mistaken for

Common thyme (*Thymus vulgaris*), which is a garden escapee, common wild thyme (*T. praecox*) and larger wild thyme (*T. pulegioides*) can all be used for the same medicinal purposes.

Where to look

Wild thyme grows in dry, well-drained soil and is often found clinging to rocky crevices and growing

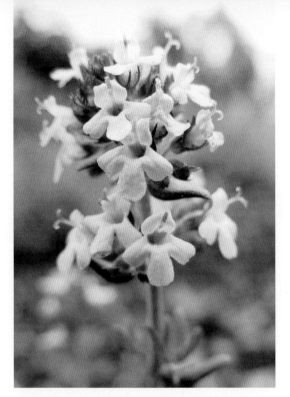

The types and concentrations of volatile oils that thymes contain differ depending on when they are grown.

Wild thyme

from seemingly soilless places. It can also be found growing in gardens.

When to look for it

Wild thyme is evergreen and flowers in June and July.

What to harvest

The whole plant.

What is it good for?

Gums and teeth • Mouth ulcers • Wounds • Asthma • Bronchitis • Catarrh • Coughs • Sore throat • Fungal infections • Infection • Bloating • Colic • Diverticular disease • Flatulence • Cystitis

Garden visitors

How to use it

Make a fresh herb tincture, which will preserve most of its volatile oils. Take this tincture in tincture blends, diluted in water for washes, or added to base creams for fungal infections. Use the dry or fresh herb as infusions for tea, for mouthwashes and gargles, for skin washes or as a vaginal douche for thrush. Use a lid when infusing it to reduce loss of volatile oils.

Cautions

Do not take in therapeutic quantities during pregnancy as the oil can stimulate the uterus.

Combines well with

Wood avens (see page 44) for sore throats and mouths
Mint (see page 198) for colic and flatulence
Elecampane (see page 140) for coughs with copious mucus
Fumitory (see page 99) as a skin wash for infections
Agrimony (see page 87) for diverticulitis
Mullein (see page 158) for dry coughs and asthma

Try it in thyme cough candy

This tasty cough candy provides excellent relief from dry, tickly coughs and sore throat. Infuse 25 g (1 oz) dried thyme herb in 400 ml (14 fl oz) water. Strain and press out all the liquid. For every 200 ml (7 fl oz) of liquid, add 300 g (10 oz) soft brown sugar. Stir until dissolved over the heat, then bring to the boil. Add 1 heaped teaspoon butter. Maintain a gentle boil until the syrup sets into a hard ball when a little is dropped into cold water. The boiling process to reach setting point may take some time. Pour into a buttered baking pan. When cool, score into 1.5 cm (3/4 in) squares. Break up when set hard, and store in a jar in the

Forager's checklist

✳ **Evergreen herb**
✳ **Widely distributed**
✳ **Grows in well-drained soil**
✳ **Small plant with a creeping habit**
✳ **Loved by bees**
✳ **Antiseptic**
✳ **10–15 cm (4–6 in) high and 30 cm (12 in) wide**
✳ **Family: Labiatae**

refrigerator. Suck one every four hours for dry or tickly coughs or for a sore throat.

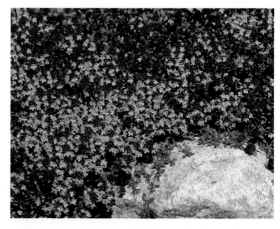

Wild thyme has a creeping habit that prefers dry conditions in full sunshine. It is easily cultivated.

Viola odorata

Sweet violet

wild violet

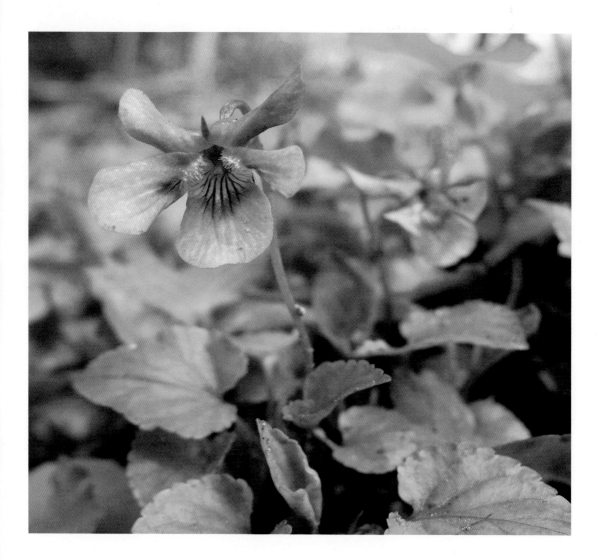

Fact and folklore

The flowers often 'hide' beneath the leaves, possibly giving rise to the term 'shrinking violet', and were traditionally crystallized and eaten as sweets to sweeten the breath. They have been used as medicine since ancient Greek times, and are mentioned in poetry and texts throughout history. The whole herb contains mucilage, which soothes inflamed mucous membranes, and saponins, which thin and break up thick mucus, so they were traditionally (and continue to be) used for coughs and sore throats. The flower syrup is a gentle laxative for children. Violet was traditionally used for treating cancers, especially of the bowel, breast and throat; records recommended drinking the infusion regularly over a long period of time. The roots are a strong purgative and emetic and best avoided.

What to look for

Sweet violet is a perennial plant that grows 10–15 cm (4–6 in) high, and has dark green, heart-shaped leaves. The flowers – sometimes hidden beneath the leaves for protection – are small, sweet scented and vary in colour from white to deep lilac. They rarely set seed because they appear before the pollinating insects do; when they do occasionally set seed and ripen, they form capsules that rise above the foliage. These seed-containing capsules have three separate sections that spring open, widely scattering the seed. The plant usually propagates itself by means of spreading underground rhizomes.

Can be mistaken for

There are many varieties of scented violet (*Viola* spp.) that all have similar medicinal properties and may all be used to treat the same conditions.

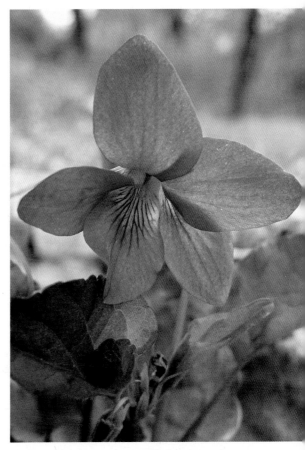

The beautiful violet imparts a wonderful colour to the syrup used for treating children's coughs and bowel problems.

Where to look

Sweet violets are found in wood margins, under large trees in parks and gardens, in hedgerows and are frequently cultivated in gardens.

When to look for it

The plant grows from January to June and flowers from March to May.

What to harvest
The whole flowering plant, and individual flowers.

What is it good for?
Catarrh • Coughs • Constipation

How to use it
Collect the flowers and make a syrup for use in constipation in children. Dry the whole plant for infusions for coughs and sore throats. Use the fresh or dried whole herb to make into a syrup to use for dry, tickly coughs and chesty coughs with thick, sticky sputum that is difficult to expectorate. Take 1–2 teaspoons up to four times a day. Tincture the whole fresh herb for use in combination with other tinctures.

Cautions
The use of this herb for cancer is by no means a cure and should only be used in conjunction with prescribed treatment from a cancer specialist and a medical herbalist. Do not use the root, which is a strong emetic and purgative.

Combines well with
Yellow dock (see page 108) for constipation
Wild thyme (see page 204), plantain (see page 105) and mullein (see page 158) for coughs
Ground ivy (see page 175) and elderflower (see page 184) for chronic catarrh

Try it in violet flower syrup
Fill a clean jar with violet flowers and cover the blossoms with boiling water. Put the lid on and leave overnight until cool. Strain out the flowers. Measure the resulting infusion. Put the violet infusion in a pan and add 150 g (5 oz) sugar for every 200 ml (7 fl oz) of liquid and a good squeeze of lemon juice. If you do not have 200 ml (7 fl oz) of liquid, reduce the quantity of sugar accordingly. Bring to the boil and simmer for a few minutes. Then put in sterilized bottles and label. Store in the refrigerator. Take 1–2 teaspoons at night for children's constipation or coughs. Syrups keep well for up to six months but discard before if it develops mould.

Forager's checklist
✻ **Rhizomatous perennial**
✻ **Widely distributed**
✻ **Sweet-scented, white to deep lilac flowers**
✻ **Frequent garden visitor**
✻ **Harvest between March and May**
✻ **Cough remedy**
✻ **10–15 cm (4–6 in) high and 20 cm (8 in) wide**
✻ **Family: Violaceae**

Sweet violet

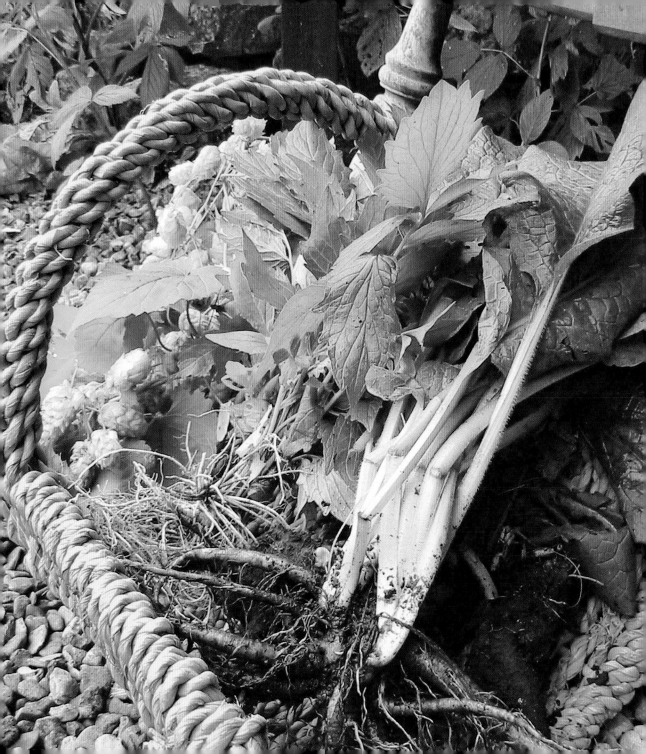

REMEDIES FOR COMMON AILMENTS

This book will give you a basic insight into the patterns of common ailments, how they arise and how herbs may help to correct the imbalance that is causing them. Try to remember that each person's body will have its own unique adaptive processes in whichever situation or environment it is in and that successful herbal treatment depends on identifying the root cause and addressing that.

The skin, eyes and mouth

Acne rosacea

This condition manifests as a bumpy, red skin rash or pimples under the skin, mainly on the nose and cheeks. It occurs predominantly in women in their 30s and 40s. Digestive dysfunction is often implicated, including sluggish liver function and gastric inflammation causing a reflex reaction in the blood vessels of the face. It is aggravated by stress, spicy food, alcohol and caffeine. Internal treatment aims to identify individual causes and rebalance hormones, heal the digestive tract and support liver function. Topical applications can help to tone and soothe inflammation.

Healing herbs

Mallow root (see page 64)
Fumitory (see page 99)
Chamomile (see page 102)
Wood betony (see page 111)
Dandelion root (see page 114)
Red clover (see page 117)
Dog rose (see page 143)
Meadowsweet (see page 169)
Daisy (see page 192)
Milk thistle (see page 195)

Treatments

❀ Take a tea of equal parts of meadowsweet, mallow and chamomile three times a day to soothe and heal the digestive tract and reduce inflammation.

❀ Add wood betony for headaches and anxiety.

❀ Add red clover if there is hormone imbalance.

❀ Use dandelion root as a tincture or coffee, or 1 teaspoon ground milk thistle seed on food to improve liver function and metabolism of hormones.

❀ An infusion of daisy can be used as a topical wash twice a day, to reduce inflammation.

Acne vulgaris

Spots that typically begin during adolescence and usually resolve within a few years, but may continue until the 30s. The symptoms are large, lumpy spots that form into heads with pus and are found on the face, back and chest. They may leave significant scarring. They are caused by hormone imbalances affecting the production of sebum and pores. It may be hereditary. Internal treatment aims to support the detoxifying systems of the liver and lymphatic systems and re-balance the hormones. Topical treatments reduce infection and reduce inflammation and scarring.

Healing herbs

Fumitory (see page 99)
Chamomile (see page 102)
Yellow dock (see page 108)
Wood Betony (see page 111)
Dandelion (see page 114)
Red clover (see page 117)
Burdock (see page 125)
Dog rose (see page 143)
Cleavers (see page 172)
Milk thistle (see page 195)

Treatments

❋ Mix 2 parts dandelion, 2 parts red clover and 1 part burdock tinctures together and take 5 ml (1 teaspoon) three times a day to improve liver function, cleanse the blood and balance hormones.

❋ Add 1 part yellow dock or 1 part fumitory if constipation is present.

❋ Take milk thistle seed tincture or 1 teaspoon ground seed if the liver is burdened with drugs or alcohol.

❋ Use an infusion of rose petals as a skin wash for antiseptic and astringent properties.

❋ Take 1 dessertspoon cleavers juice twice a day, or the tincture three times a day, to cleanse the skin via the lymph glands.

Bites and stings

Many creatures bite and sting. Some plants can also sting, nettles being the best known. They may cause a localized histamine response that can cause swelling, pain, irritation and itching. Some people are allergic and can suffer anaphylaxis, which requires emergency treatment. Herbs can provide anti-inflammatory and antihistamine effects to the area.

Healing herbs

Yarrow (see page 84)
Chamomile (see page 102)
Plantain (see page 105)

Treatments

❋ Use a bruised fresh leaf of plantain or feverfew as a poultice, changing as required. If possible, rub the plant hard between the hands and then squeeze out the juice from the leaf or flower and dab that on. Do not rub the affected area as it will aggravate the problem. Create a spit poultice by chewing a leaf.

❋ Make an ointment of infused oils of all or either yarrow, plantain and chamomile and apply it in the same way.

Boils

Caused by infections in the root of hairs, boils present initially as a painful red lump that comes up into a head and eventually discharges pus. They are usually caused by bacteria that are normally found living on the skin but take advantage of blocked pores or in-growing hairs to multiply and cause localized infections. Treatment with herbs helps to draw out pus, provide antiseptic effects and promote internal cleansing via the liver and lymphatic system. They also boost the immune system to help fight infection.

Healing herbs

Wild garlic (see page 41)
Figwort (see page 53)
Mallow root (see page 64)
Fumitory (see page 99)
Plantain (see page 105)
Burdock (see page 125)
Chickweed (see page 149)
Cleavers (see page 172)

Treatments

❋ A poultice of fresh mallow root (or moisten some dried root) and crushed wild garlic, changed every two hours, as a drawing poultice.

❋ Fresh pulverized or chewed chickweed may also be used as a drawing poultice.

❋ Fresh pulverized or chewed plantain may also be used as a drawing poultice.

❋ Eat wild garlic bulbs or leaves at least twice a day to fight the infection and boost the immune system.

❋ Take a tincture mix of 1 part burdock, 1 part figwort and 4 parts cleavers three times a day for one week to cleanse the blood and help the lymphatic system drain toxins from the skin.

❋ Add 1 part fumitory to the tincture if constipation is a problem.

Bruises

These are leakage of blood from broken blood vessels caused by a hard blow to a tissue. Localized pain, swelling and discolouration are a result, usually taking up to two weeks to resolve. Bruising can be very extensive and cause stiffness and pain if in muscles or around joints. The herbal approach aims to promote regeneration of circulation and remove damaged old blood and tissue quickly.

Healing herbs

Comfrey (see page 76)
Yarrow (see page 84)
Mugwort (see page 128)
St John's wort (see page 137)
Ground ivy (see page 175)
Daisy (see page 192)

Treatments

❋ Use an infusion or fresh bruised herb of daisy or yarrow as a compress as soon as possible to stop the bleeding.

❋ Apply comfrey or St John's wort ointment to the area three times a day to speed up the healing of the blood vessels.

❋ Use fresh bruised ground ivy as a poultice for stubborn old bruises that are slow to heal.

❋ For stubborn, old, bruises use moxa sticks (see page 130).

Burns

Burns can result from contact with hot substances, chemicals or from friction. Chemical burn treatment will be specific to the chemical and detailed on the chemical container. Burns result in redness, blistering and localized pain. Any burns larger than 7.5 cm (3 in) require medical attention, especially if they are blistered. Herbs can help to reduce pain from damaged nerves, stimulate new tissue growth and reduce the risk of infection.

Healing herbs

Comfrey (see page 76)
Yarrow (see page 84)
St John's wort (see page 137)

Treatments

❋ Put the burn under cold water for as long as possible to stop the burning, which continues after contact.

❋ If blistering is present, use infusions of yarrow and comfrey as cold compresses. Soak clean gauze or cotton in the infusion and lay gently on the burn, refreshing every hour.

❋ If there is no blistering, use St John's wort flower oil to speed healing.

Cold sores

Sores that are caused by the herpes simplex virus, which dwells in the nerve root of the spine. It takes advantage of low resistance to re-emerge. An attack is usually heralded by a tingling sensation, then a painful blister forms, which bursts and dries out, leaving a sore. They can occur anywhere on the body, but are commonly found around the mouth and on the genitals; they can be spread from one site to the other by touching, kissing and oral sex. Herpes simplex is highly contagious during the active phase. Cold sores are often precipitated by sun exposure, infection, poor diet, fatigue and poor immunity. Treatments aim to support the nerves by nourishing them and encouraging cell repair. They also provide immune stimulation to fight the infection, have an antiviral effect and promote skin healing.

Healing herbs
Wild garlic (see page 41)
Yarrow (see page 84)
Oat (see page 93)
St John's wort (see page 137)
Vervain (see page 161)
Meadowsweet (see page 169)

Treatments
❋ Take St John's wort tincture or tea every two hours for eight doses when an attack threatens for its antiviral and nerve restorative properties. After that, take four times a day until better.
❋ Include oats in the diet or take the tincture three times a day to strengthen the nerves.
❋ Eat wild garlic regularly to boost a weak immune system and for its antiviral properties.
❋ Take vervain tea up to three times a day to support the liver and nerves during and after infection.
❋ Use an ointment of meadowsweet and/or yarrow flowers every hour on the sores for their anti-inflammatory and healing properties.

Conjunctivitis
An infection of the membranes of the eyes caused by bacteria, virus or allergy. Infection gives symptoms of red, irritated eyes. Bacterial infection gives a sticky discharge, usually yellow, that can glue the eyelids together on waking. The virus is mainly associated with colds and throat infections. Infection can pass from eye to eye by contact and rubbing. Allergy causes itching and watering. Conjunctivitis often spontaneously resolves as the immune system fights the infection. Herbs help to speed up this process by being directly anti-infective and by boosting the immune system.

Healing herbs
Wild garlic (see page 41)
Eyebright (see page 96)
Chamomile (see page 102)
Dog rose petals (see page 143)
Chickweed (see page 149)
Ground ivy (see page 175)
Elderflower (see page 184)

Treatments
❋ Eat wild garlic for its anti-infectious and immune-boosting properties.
❋ Bath eyes with an infusion of equal parts of any of the above herbs every two hours during the acute stage and then three times a day until better. Use fresh infusion for each eye.

Eczema
Eczema is an allergic condition of the skin causing itching, redness, excoriation and little blisters. It may be genetic and linked with a family trait of asthma, hayfever and allergies called atopy. Seborrhoeic eczema is a dry scaling of the scalp, sides of the nose, eyebrows and ears. Contact eczema is a localized allergic response to direct contact with allergens such as hair dyes, detergents or jewellery, also known as

contact dermatitis. There is an increase in histamine in the skin and increased immune activity. It is made worse by stress, environmental pollutants, dietary additives and preservatives. A deficiency of zinc and essential fatty acids has also been implicated. Herbal approaches aim to strengthen the organs of elimination by supporting the liver and lymphatic system to remove aggravating irritants from the skin and encourage their removal from the body. This means they are flushed out via the bowels and urinary systems rather than being eliminated via the skin. Topical treatments provide a moisturizing, waterproof barrier, promote healing and reduce itching and the risk of infection. Eczema is difficult to self treat, if in doubt, consult with a medical herbalist. See Varicose veins (see page 231) for varicose eczema.

Healing herbs
Yarrow (see page 84)
Chamomile (see page 102)
Plantain (see page 105)
Yellow dock (see page 108)
Dandelion root (see page 114)
Red clover (see page 117)
Burdock (see page 125)
Chickweed (see page 149)
Nettle (see page 155)
Cleavers (see page 172)
Elderflower (see page 184)

Treatments
❋ Use chickweed and yellow dock for itching as a tincture mix of 1 part yellow dock to 4 parts chickweed. 1 teaspoon three times a day.
❋ Add burdock to the tincture in small doses very gradually to support cleansing.

❋ Take a tea of equal parts of chamomile, plantain and red clover three times a day for anti-allergenic and blood-cleansing effects.
❋ Add nettle if the eczema is wet.
❋ Add cleavers if the eczema is hot and dry or with swollen glands.
❋ Take dandelion coffee or tincture up to three times a day to strengthen the liver.

External treatments
❋ Make an ointment of infused oils of equal parts of chamomile or yarrow, chickweed and plantain. Use the ointment as required. It may also be made into an infusion from dried herbs and used in the bath or as compresses.
❋ Add elderflowers if the skin is very dry.
❋ Add comfrey infused oil if scarring is present.

Gums and teeth
Problems include gum inflammation, such as gingivitis, and tooth decay. These issues are usually caused by a high-sugar diet and poor dental hygiene, although other factors may contribute, such as smoking. Herbs can reduce infection and tone up inflamed gums, preventing bleeding and the invasion of further harmful bacteria, tartar and food particles.

Healing herbs
Wood avens (see page 44)
Oak (see page 47)
Silverweed (see page 70)
Yarrow (see page 84)
Shepherd's purse (see page 131)
Dog rose (see page 143)
Wild thyme (see page 204)

Treatments

❋ Make a mouthwash from a mixture of equal parts of any of the above herb tinctures and use 10 ml (2 teaspoons) in approximately 15 ml (1/2 fl oz) water as a mouthwash after brushing teeth twice a day.

Mouth ulcers

Painful little sores in the mouth, usually around the gums, that may occur singly or multiply when the immune system is low. They usually resolve within ten days. Herbal remedies provide pain relief and antiviral and healing properties.

Healing herbs

Wood avens (see page 44)
Silverweed (see page 70)
Yarrow (see page 84)
Wild thyme (see page 204)

Treatments

❋ Make an infusion of a mix of equal amounts of any of the above herbs and use as a mouthwash every two hours.

Psoriasis

A skin condition causing thick plaques, mainly on the extensor surfaces of the skin (knees and elbows), but it may form all over the body, including the scalp. They have clearly demarcated edges and silvery layers of skin on their surface that flake off and may bleed and crack underneath. The skin is rapidly reproducing at a much faster rate than normal. The causes are poorly understood, but it is known to be aggravated by food sensitivities and stress. Using herbs internally will help to improve elimination of immune-irritating toxins and allergens from the skin via the lymphatic system,

liver, urinary and digestive system. In times of stress they can help to soothe the nervous system and help the liver break down stress hormones. The immune system is supported and reactions can be reduced by anti-allergenic properties. Increasing the intake of essential fatty acids in the diet is also important.

Healing herbs

Figwort (see page 53)
Comfrey (see page 76)
Fumitory (see page 99)
Plantain (see page 105)
Yellow dock (see page 108)
Dandelion root (see page 114)
Red clover (see page 117)
Burdock (see page 125)
St John's wort (see page 137)
Chickweed (see page 149)
Cleavers (see page 172)
Elder (see page 184)
Milk thistle (see page 195)

Treatments

❋ Make a tincture mix of 2 parts plantain, 1 part yellow dock, 1 part burdock, 1 part figwort and 2 parts cleavers and take three times a day as a liver- and blood-cleansing, lymphatic tonic.

❋ 1 part fumitory may be used instead of yellow dock.

❋ Add 2 parts red clover if hormone imbalance is present.

❋ Add 2 parts chickweed tincture internally and use chickweed salve externally, if itching is present.

❋ Make an ointment of any of St John's wort- comfrey- elderflower- and plantain-infused oil and apply to affected areas twice a day.

❊ Drink dandelion coffee (see page 116) every day to support the liver.

❊ Take ground milk thistle seed or tincture if alcohol or drugs are an issue.

Sunburn

Caused by over-exposure of unprotected skin to the sun. On hot, sunny days it may occur within 15 minutes of sun exposure. Fair skins are more prone than olive or darker skin tones. Long-term risks of sunburn and skin damage are skin ageing and skin cancer (malignant melanoma). Topically, herbs help to draw out heat and to promote tissue repair and reduce pain.

Healing herbs
Plantain (see page 105)
St John's wort (see page 137)

Treatments
❊ Apply the juice of plantain leaves to the burns to cool and reduce inflammation.
❊ Use St John's wort-infused oil for its skin-healing properties and pain reduction.

Warts and verrucas

Both warts and verrucas are caused by the papilloma virus. A verruca is a wart on the bottom of the foot that gets pushed flat. They may spread prolifically over a small area, usually on the hands or feet. They often spontaneously resolve as the immune system becomes resistant to them. Warts and verrucas rarely cause any further problems, other than local effects of discomfort, and are disfiguring on the hands. Genital warts, however, have been linked with increased risk of cervical cancer.

Healing herbs
Dandelion (see page 114)
Celandine (see page 134)

Treatments
❊ Apply the sap of either plant to the wart or verruca, every day for at least a month or until it peels off. Do not get the sap on the surrounding skin. Only treat a few warts at a time. It is not advised to treat genital or facial warts with this remedy.

Wounds

Cuts, sores and grazes that bleed (see Bleeding, page 228), cause pain and take time to heal. Infection may be a complication. Many herbs have excellent properties that promote tissue regrowth and reduce the risk of infection.

Healing herbs
Comfrey (see page 76)
Yarrow (see page 84)
Plantain (see page 105)
St John's wort (see page 137)
Wild thyme (see page 204)

Treatments
❊ For open wounds, use an infusion of comfrey as a wash.
❊ For wounds that have scabbed over, use an ointment of any of the above herbs for their healing properties.
❊ Use an infusion of wild thyme as a wash if infection threatens.
❊ Beware of using comfrey on deep wounds, as it heals so quickly it has been known to cause a wound to heal over the top, leaving a cavity underneath.

The musculo-skeletal system

Arthritis

Degeneration of the joint internal surfaces causing pain, stiffness and restricted movement. It is usually seen in weight-bearing joints of knees and hips, but also in wrists, fingers, base of the thumb and spine. It is common in elderly, menopausal women and in joints that have sustained injury throughout life. Possible mechanisms are digestive disturbance and inefficient routes of elimination leading to accumulation of toxins in the joint spaces. The immune system tries to 'tidy up' causing inflammation. This then heals, causing scarring of the cartilage and bony overgrowth at the edges of the joints that appear as deformities.

Healing herbs

Horsetail (see page 67)
Willow bark (see page 73)
Comfrey (see page 76)
Dandelion root (see page 114)
Horseradish (see page 122)
Burdock (see page 125)
Nettle (see page 155)
Meadowsweet (see page 169)
Daisy (see page 192)
Feverfew (see page 201)

Treatments

✳ Take nettle tea or dandelion coffee (see page 116) three times a day, and include in the diet for their joint-cleansing and eliminative properties.
✳ Use horsetail tincture or tea for its joint restorative mineral content.
✳ Use burdock root tincture to support the liver and cleanse the system.
✳ Take meadowsweet tincture three times a day for anti-inflammatory and digestive healing effects. Alternatively, take willow bark or feverfew tincture three times a day for anti-inflammatory effects.
✳ Take daisy tincture for blood and joint cleansing.
✳ Use comfrey, meadowsweet or horseradish ointment twice a day over the affected area to facilitate tissue repair and stimulate circulation.

Backache

This may occur anywhere on the back but is most commonly experienced in the lower lumbar region. It may be caused by muscle strain, poor abdominal and core muscle strength, poor posture, or disc and vertebral problems. Exercise, posture correction and improving core muscle strength are all effective, long-term treatments. Kidney, bladder, bowel, menstrual and ovarian conditions may all refer pain into the lower half of the back. The liver and gall bladder, lungs and oesophagus may all refer pain into the upper half.

Healing herbs

Comfrey (see page 76)
Valerian (see page 79)
Horseradish (see page 122)
St John's wort (see page 137)
Cramp bark (see page 187)

Treatments

❋ Take 10 ml (2 teaspoons) of a mix of equal parts of valerian and hop tincture twice a day if muscle spasm is present.

❋ Use an ointment of horseradish and use twice a day on the affected area for healing and to improve circulation.

❋ Massage in a liniment of equal parts St John's wort-infused oil and cramp bark tincture to relax and relieve muscle spasm.

❋ If nerve pain is present, take St John's wort tincture three times a day to restore the nerves.

Cramp

A painful, prolonged contraction of the muscles, usually of the calf, but it may occur in any muscle of the body. Cramp is caused by an imbalance of the blood electrolytes – calcium, magnesium, potassium and sodium – from excessive sweating during exercise or pregnancy and, more rarely, multiple sclerosis and kidney disease. Cramp may also be due to medications such as diuretics and statins. Other risk factors include hypothyroidism, reduced blood flow (see Atherosclerosis, page 227) and extreme changes in temperature. Women are more prone than men.

Healing herbs

Wild garlic (see page 41)
Valerian (see page 79)
Oat (see page 93)
Chamomile (see page 102)
Horseradish (see page 122)
Cramp bark (see bark 187)

Treatments

❋ Take 10 ml (2 teaspoons) of either valerian root or cramp bark tincture for its relaxing effects; it is also rich in calcium.

❋ Include nettles, horseradish and oats in the diet for their rich electrolyte content.

❋ Massage infused oil of chamomile or cramp bark liniment into the affected area to relieve a cramp.

❋ Include wild garlic in the diet to improve circulation.

Gout

Excruciating pain and inflammation of the joints, usually of the big toe, that is caused by deposits of uric acid crystals as a result of faulty protein metabolism and elimination. Signs are tight, red, shiny skin over the affected area. It is more common in men and aggravated by a diet rich in animal proteins.

Healing herbs

Willow bark (see page 73)
Couch grass (see page 90)
Dandelion root (see page 114)
Burdock (see page 125)
Nettle (see page 155)
Meadowsweet (see page 169)
Daisy (see page 192)
Milk thistle (see page 195)

Treatments

❋ Drink nettle tea three times a day to dissolve and eliminate the acid.

❋ Drink dandelion coffee (see page 116) three times a day to support the liver.

❋ Take milk thistle or burdock tincture to improve liver function.

❋ Take meadowsweet and willow tincture three times a day for their anti-inflammatory effects.

❋ Drink couch grass tea to improve removal of waste products via the kidneys and urinary tract.

❋ Take daisy tincture for its blood-cleansing effects.

Osteoporosis

Also known as brittle bone disease, osteoporosis is caused by demineralization of the bones, causing weakness. The bones fracture easily and the spine can compress as the vertebrae collapse. Women are more prone than men, because after menopause they no longer benefit from the bone-protecting effects of oestrogen. Risk factors are high alcohol intake, anorexia, premature menopause (natural or surgical) and a low-calcium diet.

Healing herbs
Horsetail (see page 67)
Comfrey (see page 76)
Oat (see page 93)
Nettle (see page 155)

Treatments
❋ Drink nettle tea three times a day for the rich mineral content.

❋ Take 1 dessertspoon horsetail juice twice a day for the bone-strengthening silica.

❋ Take oat tincture three times a day for its nutrient-rich content, and eat the groats regularly.

❋ Use comfrey topically for fractures, and take the infusion internally for short periods.

Restless leg syndrome

A distressing condition characterized by twitchy legs, especially at night. It is most commonly seen in women and the elderly. Anaemia, pregnancy, chronic diseases and medications may aggravate it.

Healing herbs
Lime (see page 56)
Valerian (see page 79)
Oat (see page 93)
Chamomile (see page 102)
St John's wort (see page 137)
Cramp bark (see page 187)

Treatments
❋ Take a mix of equal parts St John's wort, oats and limeflower tinctures three times a day.

❋ Make a tincture mix of equal parts hops and valerian and take up to 15 ml ($^1/_2$ fl oz) at night for sleep.

❋ Massage the calf muscles with liniment of 2 parts chamomile-infused oil and 1 part tincture of cramp bark or valerian every evening before bed.

Sprains and strains

A sprain is an over-stretch or tear of a ligament, which is a tough band of tissue that joins one bone to another, and a strain is an over-stretch or tear of a muscle or tendon. Tendons join muscles to bones.

Healing herbs
Comfrey (see page 76)
Horseradish (see page 122)
Meadowsweet (see page 169)
Daisy (see page 192)

Treatments
❋ Apply a poultice of comfrey root or leaf as soon as possible, and renew it every two hours.

❋ Use an infusion of daisy as a cold compress, changing it every hour for the rest of the day.

❋ Massage in 2 parts comfrey and 1 part horseradish-infused oil or as an ointment twice a day.

The musculo-skeletal system

The respiratory system

Asthma

A distressing respiratory condition causing shortness of breath and wheezing. It is often a combination of causes, including allergy, anxiety, hyperventilation, chronic mouth breathing and inherited factors. Sufferers can have an increased risk of respiratory tract infection, usually as a complication of viral infections. It is aggravated by exercise, cold, allergens, stress and infection. Inhaled bronchodilators can save lives.

Healing herbs
Mallow (see page 64)
Elecampane (see page 140)
Coltsfoot (see page 152)
Mullein (see page 158)
Wild thyme (see page 204)

Treatments
❋ Take a tea of equal parts mullein, coltsfoot and marsh mallow up to six times a day to reduce spasm and relieve dry coughs and wheezing.
❋ Take elecampane and thyme tincture up to six times a day for infections with lots of mucus.
❋ 'Buteyko breathing' (named after the Russian doctor who developed it, Konstantin Buteyko) has been shown to reduce asthma symptoms significantly (see www.buteykobreathing.org for details).

Bronchitis

A chronic cough and infection, with copious, thick, sticky mucus and inflammation of the lungs. People who get bronchitis regularly usually have some form of chronic lung disease. For them, it often occurs as a secondary complication of a minor viral or bacterial infection of the upper respiratory tract like a cold or sore throat.

Healing herbs
Wild garlic (see page 41)
Mallow (see page 64)
Horseradish (see page 122)
Elecampane (see page 140)
Coltsfoot (see page 152)
Mullein (see page 158)
Wild thyme (see page 204)

Treatments
❋ Take 1 teaspoon of elecampane syrup three times a day as a lung restorative and for its antibacterial properties.
❋ For very thick, sticky mucus that is hard to expectorate, add mallow, mullein or coltsfoot to thin it and ease its passage.
❋ Include horseradish in the diet or take 1 teaspoon of the syrup three times a day to stimulate expectoration.
❋ Eat raw wild garlic or take wild garlic honey three times a day for its deep antibacterial action and to liquefy mucus.
❋ Drink thyme tea up to three times a day to promote expectoration and for its antispasmodic and antibacterial properties.

Catarrh

Often manifests as a chronic condition following colds, or as a result of allergic rhinitis. It is an excessive discharge of mucus from the mucous membranes of the sinuses, throat and upper respiratory tract. It is caused by inflammation of the mucous membranes and the symptoms are blocked, congested nose, post-nasal drip, throat clearing and cough. There are often associated food sensitivities; dairy products are often blamed as they can increase mucus production.

Healing herbs

Wild garlic (see page 41)
Oak (see page 47)
Eyebright (see page 96)
Horeseradish (see page 122)
Elecampane (see page 140)
Golden rod (see page 146)
Mullein (see page 158)
Ground ivy (see page 175)
Elderflower (see page 184)
Mint (see page 198)
Wild thyme (see page 204)
Sweet violet (see page 207)

Treatments

✻ Drink a tea of equal amounts of any of the following herbs: ground ivy, eyebright, elderflower, violet and golden rod three times a day for their mucous membrane tonic effects.
✻ Add mint for its decongestant effects.
✻ Take elecampane syrup three times a day for mucus in the throat and lungs. It will warm and dry up 'boggy' mucous membranes.
✻ Add wild thyme, wild garlic or horseradish if infection is present.

✻ Take a tiny pinch of powdered oak bark as a snuff twice a day for streaming mucus from the nose, or for nasal polyps, to astringe and tone the mucous membranes.

Colds

Colds are caused by various different strains of rhinoviruses, 'rhino' coming from the Greek for nose. They are the most common virus affecting humans. The main symptoms are itchy, runny and congested nose, sore throat, sneezing and cough. They are spread by airborne droplets (sneezing) and by contact with a contaminated surface. A saying about colds goes: 'Three days coming, three days staying, three days going.' There is often a secondary bacterial infection taking advantage of a weakened state and the inflamed mucous membranes.

Healing herbs

Wild garlic (see page 41)
Yarrow (see page 84)
Dog rose (see page 143)
Golden rod (see page 146)
Ground ivy (see page 175)
Elder (see page 184)
Mint (see page 198)

Treatments

✻ Take an infusion of a combination of equal amounts of elderflower, peppermint and yarrow. Drink 1 pint (600 ml), hot, at the first sign and go to bed to halt the infection. Continue drinking this tea until better.
✻ Take elderberry syrup or tincture every two hours for eight doses, and then three times a day until better for its antiviral effects.

The respiratory system

✻ Use rosehip syrup for its immune-boosting vitamin C content.

✻ Eat wild garlic for its anti-infective properties.

✻ Take equal amounts of ground ivy and golden rod as a tea, or alternatively as a tincture, for mucous membrane congestion.

Coughs

Dry, tickly coughs are a sign of inflamed mucous membranes of the respiratory tract. They happen as a result of viral or bacterial infection and often follow colds when mouth breathing is depended on because the nose is blocked. Whooping cough is called the 'hundred day cough' in Chinese medicine and is caused by a virus. Both of these need mucilaginous herbs to soothe and reduce inflammation. Phlegmy coughs require stimulation with expectorant herbs to loosen and expel mucous. If the phlegm becomes chronic use mucus membrane tonics to restore the tone of the membranes lining the airways and reduce mucus production.

Healing herbs

For dry coughs:

Limeflower (see page 56)

Mallow (see page 64)

Plantain (see page 105)

Coltsfoot (see page 152)

Mullein (see page 158)

Wild thyme (see page 204)

Sweet violet (see page 207)

For mucous coughs:

Wild garlic (see page 41)

Horseradish (see page 122)

Elecampane (see page 140)

Ground ivy (see page 175)

Wild thyme (see page 204)

Sweet violet (see page 207)

Treatments

✻ For dry coughs, take a combination of equal amounts of any of the herbs listed as a tea, sipping freely. Alternatively, make a tincture and take every two hours for an acute cough and three times a day for chronic coughs.

✻ For mucous coughs, follow the directions given for bronchitis (see page 222).

Earache

This usually derives from infection, causing otitis externa (outer ear infection) or otitis media (middle ear infection). Outer ear infections cause visible redness and inflammation and localized pain and discharge. They are often picked up when swimming and can also be introduced by a scratch from a nail. Middle ear infections occur behind the eardrum. They can cause pain, malaise, deafness and sometimes dizziness. They are often spread from infections of the nose or throat via the Eustachian tube. Young children often suffer with a condition called glue ear, a catarrh problem that causes a thick build up of secretions in the middle ear. Earache may also be caused by problems with the teeth and jaw.

Healing herbs

Wild garlic (see page 41)

Yarrow (see page 84)

Chamomile (see page 102)

Plantain (see page 105)

Mullein (see page 158)

Ground ivy (see page 175)

Treatments

❁ Combine equal amounts of infused oils of mullein and chamomile flowers as eardrops, and apply 6 drops every four hours. For otitis externa, also massage this oil around the outside of the ear.

❁ Tie a small piece of wild garlic bulb in a piece of muslin and put this just inside the ear canal overnight, ensuring it can be pulled out in the morning. Alternatively, make garlic-infused oil by chopping three bulbs of garlic and covering it with sunflower oil overnight; strain and use as eardrops – 4 drops every four hours. (Do not do both.)

❁ Take tea or tinctures of equal amounts of plantain, yarrow and ground ivy every four hours to tone the mucous membranes and boost the immune system.

Flu (influenza)

There are many strains of influenza virus. Flu is a severe viral infection, causing sore throat, headache, muscle aches, weakness, fever and cough. It is extremely debilitating and patients are bed-bound for at least a week; it is often two weeks before people recover. Secondary infection, such as pneumonia, is a common complication, particularly in the elderly or those with lowered immunity. It is contagious and spread by droplet infection.

Healing herbs

Wild garlic (see page 41)
Yarrow (see page 84)
Dog rose (see page 143)
Elder (see page 184)
Mint (see page 198)

Treatments

❁ Take wild garlic honey for any cough and sore throat symptoms.

❁ Take 1 teaspoon elderberry syrup, tincture or compound in water every two hours for eight doses, and then four times a day until better.

❁ Take rosehip syrup for its immune-boosting vitamin C content.

❁ Drink a hot infusion of equal amounts of elderflower, mint and yarrow freely throughout the illness to reduce fever, chills and aching.

❁ Take white willow tincture for severe joint and muscle aching.

Hayfever

Also known as seasonal rhinitis, hayfever is caused by hypersensitivity to tree, grass and flower pollens and fungal spores. The symptoms include itchy nose, eyes and throat, watering eyes, runny or congested nose and sneezing, as a result of excess histamine production. It starts in the spring and can last until autumn. People may be allergic to just one or many different pollens. Perennial rhinitis is experienced all year round. The herbal approach is to regulate the immune system and use mucous membrane tonics.

Healing herbs

Eyebright (see page 96)
Chamomile (see page 102)
Plantain (see page 105)
Golden rod (see page 146)
Nettle (see page 155)
Ground ivy (see page 175)
Elderflower (see page 184)

Treatments

❁ Make a combination tincture of equal amounts of nettle, elderflower, eyebright, plantain and ground ivy and take 2 teaspoons twice a day. Start taking the tincture at least six weeks before the symptoms normally emerge.

❋ Make a fresh infusion daily of equal parts eyebright and chamomile. Strain through a fine muslin and use the infusion as an eyebath twice a day for itching and irritation.

Sinusitis

Infection and congestion of the sinuses, usually as a complication of a cold. Sinusitis causes pain, headaches, blocked nose, loss of smell and thick mucus, which is usually yellow or green.

Healing herbs
Wild garlic (see page 41)
Horseradish (see page 122)
Elecampane (see page 140)
Ground ivy (see page 175)
Elderflower (see page 184)
Mint (see page 198)

Treatments
❋ Eat wild garlic leaves and bulbs three times a day to beat the infection.
❋ Take horseradish syrup, to stimulate the circulation in the sinuses. Alternatively, eat the syrup as a condiment with food.
❋ Take elecampane honey up to every two hours for its decongestant, antiseptic effects.
❋ Drink a hot infusion of equal amounts of any of ground ivy, golden rod, mint and elderflower up to six times a day to reduce congestion and tone the mucous membranes of the nose.
❋ Use a warm infusion of ground ivy (see page 175) as a nasal douche every few hours.

Sore throat

Sore throats are usually caused by viral infections. The throat and tonsils are red and there is pain on swallowing. The tonsils may become very enlarged – this is known as tonsillitis. A sore throat may develop as a complication of a cold. The lymph glands in the neck may be enlarged in all cases.

Healing herbs
Wild garlic (see page 41)
Wood avens (see page 44)
Oak (see page 47)
Limeflower (see page 56)
Mallow (see page 64)
Silverweed (see page 70)
Yarrow (see page 84)
Shepherd's purse (see page 131)
Elecampane (see page 140)
Elderberry (see page 184)
Cleavers (see page 172)
Wild thyme (see page 204)

Treatments
❋ Eat wild garlic leaves and bulbs on toast or honey for powerful anti-infective effects.
❋ Take elderberry tincture or syrup every two hours for eight doses, and then four times a day until better.
❋ Gargle and swallow tea or tincture of equal amounts wood avens, mallow and wild thyme every four hours.
❋ Take a teaspoon of limeflower or elecampane honey every two hours for their antiseptic properties.
❋ Take cleavers juice or tincture three times a day for swollen glands.
❋ Gargle with silverweed, shepherds purse or oak bark tincture or infusion after the infection, if the tonsils are chronically enlarged, to tone them.

Anaemia

This is characterized by low haemoglobin and reduced red blood cells. It is caused by bleeding, reduced red blood cell production, low iron levels, increased destruction of red blood cells by the spleen and inability to absorb vitamin B12 and folic acid. The symptoms are shortness of breath and fatigue, and the signs are pale mucous membranes inside the lips and eyelids, as well as general pallor. Look to improve digestive function and absorption of iron and vitamin C. Take herbs that are easily absorbed and rich in iron, vitamins and minerals.

Healing herbs

Oat (see page 93)
Yellow dock (see page 108)
Shepherd's purse (see page 131)
Chickweed (see page 149)
Nettle (see page 155)

Treatments

❋ Eat nettles every day in soups and stews, or cooked as a vegetable, for their rich vitamin, mineral and iron content.

❋ Drink equal amounts of nettle and chickweed tea three times a day; they are both rich in iron.

❋ Take yellow dock tincture once a day to improve digestion and bowel health; it is also rich in iron.

❋ Look for the cause of the anaemia and apply appropriate herbs to treat. For example, for bleeding use astringent herbs such as shepherd's purse.

Atherosclerosis

Atherosclerosis is the build-up of fatty deposits on the inside of the arterial walls, which leads to arteriosclerosis, a thickening, stiffening and loss of elasticity of the arteries. It causes restricted blood flow and increases pressure in the arteries. It increases the risk of high blood pressure, angina, heart attacks, circulation problems and strokes. Risk factors include smoking, diabetes, stress and a diet that is high in hydrogenated and trans fatty acids and low in fruit and vegetables. It is also hereditary. Herbs that are rich in flavonoids help to improve the health of the blood vessel walls and reduce the inflammation that causes the deposits of fats. Relaxant herbs reduce stress and relax the smooth muscle surrounding the blood vessels. Appropriate herbs also encourage the production of beneficial, high density, lipo proteins.

Healing herbs

Wild garlic (see page 41)
Limeflower (see page 56)
Dandelion root (see page 114)
Hawthorn (see page 166)
Milk thistle (see page 195)

Treatments

❋ Take wild garlic every day in the diet for its heart and blood vessel protective effects.

❋ Take limeflower tea three times a day for its flavonoids, which help improve blood vessel health.

❋ Take a tincture of hawthorn three times a day for

its heart and blood vessel tonic effects.

❋ Take dandelion root or milk thistle as a tincture or as dandelion coffee (see page 116) or ground milk thistle seed to support the liver and improve digestion of fats.

Bleeding

This normally occurs as a result of trauma, wounds, inflammation or infection. Heavy menstrual bleeding (see page 246) is usually a result of hormone imbalance or fibroids. It may also arise from clotting disorders or as a result of blood thinning medications. Cancer may also cause unusual bleeding. Different areas of the body indicates different herbs that have an affinity for that area. Bleeding may cause anaemia (see page 227). Astringent herbs close up weak and leaking capillaries to help stop bleeding. Iron and nutrient-rich herbs enable the body to replace lost red blood cells.

Healing herbs
Oak (see page 47)
Silverweed (see page 70)
Yarrow (see page 84)
Plantain (see page 105)
Shepherd's purse (see page 131)
Dog rose petals (see page 143)
Nettle (see page 155)

Treatments
❋ Apply pressure and elevate as first aid for traumatic wounds.
❋ Use fresh bruised yarrow or shepherd's purse as styptics for wounds in the field.
❋ For bleeding of the urinary tract or womb, take shepherd's purse or dog rose petals as an infusion or tincture three times a day.
❋ If you find there is bleeding of the digestive system, make a tincture of 2 parts plantain, 2 parts silverweed and 1 part oak bark. Take this tincture three times a day.
❋ For bleeding haemorrhoids (piles), (see page 230), apply compresses of equal parts of oak bark decoction and pilewort infusion.
❋ Drink nettle tea up to three times a day for bleeding anywhere on the body, to provide iron, vitamins and minerals.

Chilblains

A painful and irritating condition of the blood vessels of the extremities. It is triggered by cold, damp weather that causes constriction of the blood vessels, which are then warmed too quickly. The small vessels do not dilate quickly enough and the returning blood flow is forced into the tissues, causing irritation, itching, burning and redness. Young women seem to be at greatest risk. Nerve and circulatory tonic herbs help to stabilize the body's blood flow and prevent constriction. Anti-inflammatory and tissue-healing herbs speed recovery and ease symptoms.

Healing herbs
Wild garlic (see page 41)
Lime (see page 56)
Yarrow (see page 84)
Horseradish (see page 122)
Hawthorn (see page 166)
Cramp bark (see page 187)

Treatments
❋ Include wild garlic in the daily diet to improve blood flow through small vessels.

✻ Take a tea of equal parts of limeflower and hawthorn tops up to three times a day for their restorative effects on blood vessel walls.

✻ Take a tincture of cramp bark as a preventative during times when the weather increases risk of chilblains occurring.

✻ Use yarrow- or horseradish-infused oil or ointment on chilblains that are causing problems and discomfort, to stimulate circulation and reduce inflammation.

Cholesterol, high

Raised blood cholesterol is thought to be responsible for atheroma, or furring of the arteries, which increases the risk of heart disease. Raised total cholesterol levels are not a good indication of the potential problems of high cholesterol, however; they should be split into measurements of 'good' cholesterol or high-density lipoproteins (HDL) and 'bad' cholesterol or low-density lipoproteins (LDL). HDL has been shown to be protective against heart disease and LDL increases the risks of heart and blood vessel disease. The liver binds cholesterol to proteins to make these lipoproteins and enable it to be soluble in the blood and transported around the body. High cholesterol may be hereditary, and risk factors include a diet high in refined carbohydrates and hydrogenated and trans fatty acids found in processed foods. Herbal treatment aims to improve the liver function and reduce stress levels. Stress contributes to inflammation in the blood vessels. Inflammation increases the risk of cholesterol build-up on the vessel wall.

Healing herbs
Wild garlic (see page 41)

Lime (see page 56)
Oat (see page 93)
Dandelion root (see page 114)
Hawthorn (see page 166)
Milk thistle (see page 195)

Treatments
✻ Include wild garlic in the diet every day or take the tincture three times a day.

✻ Take limeflower tea three times a day for the blood vessel restorative effects and reduce the impact of stress.

✻ Take a tincture mix of equal parts milk thistle and hawthorn berry to improve liver function and protect the heart.

✻ Drink dandelion coffee (see page 116) on a daily basis to support liver function.

✻ Include oats regularly in the diet. Alternatively, take them as a tincture to help support the nervous system.

Glands, enlarged

Enlarged lymph glands can be felt in the neck, armpits and groin. They become enlarged in response to infection and inflammation, when the immune system is activated. The lymph glands can become chronically enlarged in chronic diseases of the immune system such as recurrent tonsillitis, ME, inflammatory joint, muscle and skin disease, lupus and immune system cancers.

Healing herbs
Red clover (see page 117)
Cleavers (see page 172)

Treatments

❋ Take 1 dessertspoon cleavers juice three times a day, or fresh tincture of cleavers three times a day, to assist in draining the glands of accumulated toxins.

❋ Drink the infusion of red clover tea three times a day as a lymph cleanser.

❋ Drink dandelion coffee (see page 116) to support liver function.

Haemorrhoids (piles)

Piles are inflamed veins in and around the anus that present as little, grape-like protrusions; they are painful, sore and itchy, and may bleed (see Bleeding, page 228). Piles indicate pelvic blood congestion, and the commonest causes are constipation, straining and pregnancy. (If varicose veins are present, see Varicose veins, page 231.) Astringent herbs internally tone up the veins, reducing engorgement. Externally, they are directly soothing and speed the healing of the vessels.

Healing herbs

Horse chestnut (page 38)
Oak (see page 47)
Pilewort (see page 50)
Silverweed (see page 70)
Yarrow (see page 84)
Shepherd's purse (see page 131)
Daisy (see page 192)

Treatments

❋ Use pilewort ointment three times a day.

❋ Use a compress of infusions of equal amounts of silverweed or oak bark and horse chestnut. Alternatively, make an ointment of equal amounts of horse chestnut and yarrow and use three times a day (see page 40). (Do not use both.)

❋ Make a tea of equal amounts of yarrow and shepherd's purse. Drink this three times a day to improve the pelvic blood flow and for their anti-inflammatory effects.

❋ Take horse chestnut tincture twice a day as a venous tonic.

High blood pressure

High blood pressure is a symptom, not a condition. Blood pressure is a measurement of the maximum pressure the heart exerts to pump the blood through the blood vessels and the minimum pressure the blood vessels are at under rest, between heart beats. This is expressed as two figures, for example 120/70. The higher number is a measure of the 'systolic' pressure, when the heart is contracting, and the lower number is a measure of the 'diastolic' pressure when the heart is between contractions. High blood pressure (usually defined as 140/90 or above) often shows no symptoms except, rarely, headaches; complications are heart attack and stroke. Its causes are often not understood, but stress and anxiety, smoking and kidney disease are known to be factors. Herbs address stress, relax the mind and smooth muscles surrounding the arteries. They also improve blood vessel health.

Healing herbs

Wild garlic (see page 41)
Lime (see page 56)
Mistletoe (see page 59)
Valerian (see page 79)
Yarrow (see page 84)
Dandelion (see page 114)
Hawthorn (see page 166)
Cramp bark (see page 187)

Treatments

❊ Drink limeflower tea three times a day to restore and relax the blood vessel walls.

❊ Take a tincture of 2 parts hawthorn, 2 parts yarrow, 1 part cramp bark and 1 part mistletoe three times a day to restore the blood vessels and relax the artery walls.

❊ Add wood betony if headache is present.

❊ Add valerian if stress and anxiety are factors.

❊ Eat wild garlic every day for its heart-protective effects.

Nosebleed

This condition may be recurrent, resulting from inflamed blood vessels or infections (see Sinusitis, page 225), as a result of trauma including nose-blowing, or as a side-effect of blood-thinning medications or high blood pressure.

Healing herbs

Oak (see page 47)
Silverweed (see page 70)
Yarrow (see page 84)
Shepherd's purse (see page 131)

Treatments

❊ For frequent nosebleeds, try a tiny pinch of powdered oak bark as a snuff every morning for two weeks to close a leaky blood vessel.

❊ To halt a nosebleed, dilute 1 teaspoon shepherd's purse, silverweed or yarrow tincture in a little water, soak a piece of cotton or gauze with it, and insert it up the nostril or use as nosedrops. Do not blow the nose; apply continuous pressure on the soft area towards the top of the nose and let the head drop forward until the nosebleed stops.

Varicose veins

These occur when the valves in the veins, commonly in the legs, become weak and are unable to close properly, allowing backflow and pooling of blood in the vessels below. A varicocele is a varicose vein in the testicle. Haemorrhoids are also varicose veins. Normally hidden veins become visible as lumpy, blue, tortuous veins. They may cause no symptoms but can ache, burn and itch. Varicose (or stasis) eczema may be a complication. Varicose veins are caused by reduced blood flow and increased pressure in the veins, due to inactivity, crossing the legs, pregnancy and obesity.

Healing herbs

Horse chestnut (see page 38)
Oak (see page 47)
Lime (see page 56)
Comfrey (see page 76)
Yarrow (see page 84)

Treatments

❊ Take tincture of horse chestnut twice a day to tone the veins.

❊ Drink a tea of limeflower three times a day for its blood vessel restorative effects.

❊ Use comfrey salve if there is dry skin surrounding varicose eczema.

❊ Use a lotion of yarrow, oak bark and horse chestnut twice a day on the veins.

The nervous system

Anxiety and stress

This is usually caused by over-busy lifestyles, hectic schedules, life-changing events that give no time for rest and relaxation, and pressure to perform at work and home. It manifests as perpetual worrying, insomnia, low mood, irritability and various physical ailments. A tendency to chronic anxiety and stress is said to run in families and has both genetic and learned traits. Many herbs have effects on the central nervous system, reducing tension and promoting relaxation. They reduce the sympathetic 'flight or fight' adrenaline reflexes and increase the restorative effects of the parasympathetic nervous system. Other herbs have nourishing and restorative properties that provide essential nutrients for healthy functioning.

Healing herbs

Lime (see page 56)
Valerian (see page 79)
Oat (see page 93)
Chamomile (see page 102)
Wood betony (see page 111)
St John's wort (see page 137)
Vervain (see page 161)
Hop (see page 178)

Treatments

❋ Eat oats daily as porridge, muesli, oatcakes, and so on, or take oat tincture three times a day, to provide nourishment for the nerves.
❋ Make a tea of equal amounts of chamomile and limeflower. Drink the tea three times a day to help aid relaxation.
❋ Take 1–3 teaspoons valerian tincture in water at bedtime to aid sleep, or sip it for a panic attack.
❋ Use equal amounts of St John's wort and vervain tincture three times a day if anxiety and depression are present.
❋ Add wood betony if headaches are a problem.
❋ Add hop if stress is causing irritable bowel; be aware of their depressive effects.

Chickenpox and shingles

These illnesses are caused by the varicella virus, which is similar to the herpes virus. Chickenpox usually manifests in childhood as a mild illness causing cold-like symptoms, and then itchy blister-like spots anywhere on the body. It lasts up to two weeks. The virus then retreats into the nerve root and stays dormant there. It may recur at any time as shingles, which presents as a feverish illness with a painful rash and blisters along a specific area of the skin. This distribution is allied directly to an area served by a sensory nerve, called a dermatome.

If you have had chickenpox, you cannot catch shingles from someone else with the disease. If you have not had chickenpox, you can catch it from someone with shingles. Chickenpox manifests as a more serious illness with increasing age. Chickenpox is highly contagious, spread by droplet infection from the blister fluid. When the spots are all dry, it is no longer contagious.

Healing herbs

Yarrow (see page 84)
Oat (see page 93)
Chamomile (see page 102)
St John's wort (see page 137)
Chickweed (see page 149)
Elder (see page 184)

Treatments

- Take a tea of equal parts of elderflower and yarrow for the cold symptoms and to increase sweating and natural cooling. Drink freely.
- Take St John's wort as a tincture or tea up to six times a day for its antiviral properties.
- Take elderberry tincture or syrup every 2–4 hours for its antiviral properties.
- Use equal amounts of chamomile, chickweed and St John's wort infusion as cold compresses, or the infused oil topically on the spots, for their anti-inflammatory and anti-itch properties.
- Take oat tincture for convalescence to strengthen the nerves.

Depression

Feelings of prolonged low mood with a wide range of symptoms and emotions including tearfulness, fatigue, insomnia, desire to sleep too much, lack of motivation, negative self-image, diminished joy in daily life, inability to concentrate, preoccupation about death and weight loss or gain. It may be in response to a life trauma (reactive depression), genetically predisposed (an inherited trait), psychological (caused by emotional and mental abuse) or environmental (caused by lifestyle and diet). It manifests in many different ways and may have more than one cause. It requires professional help and support. Herbal medicines can provide useful daily support for sufferers by nourishing and restoring exhausted and dysfunctioning nerves.

Healing herbs

Oat (see page 93)
Wood betony (see page 111)
Dandelion root (see page 114)
St John's wort (see page 137)
Vervain (see page 161)

Treatments

- Eat oats daily to feed the nervous system.
- Take St John's wort as a tea or tincture as a nerve restorative. Do not take in combination with orthodox drugs, or cease taking prescribed medications, without support.
- Take equal parts vervain and wood betony tincture up to three times a day to support the liver and the nerves.
- Drink dandelion coffee (see page 116) as a bitter tonic to help the liver eliminate depressive waste products from the body.

Exhaustion

This is usually caused by over-work or prolonged stress, illness or sheer physical exertion. Symptoms are fatigue, both mental and physical – the body has used all its energy reserves and cannot go on. The adrenal glands are often depleted and vital nutrients are deficient. Rest and good nutrition with diet and herbs are required for the body to restock vital reserves.

Healing herbs

Oat (see page 93)
Dog rose hips (see page 143)

Nettle (see page 155)
Vervain (see page 161)

Treatments

❊ Take 1 dessertspoon nettle seed every day, on food, to restore the adrenal glands.

❊ Put 1 dessertspoon rose hip syrup on food, or drink the tea, up to three times a day for the rich vitamin content and adrenal restorative effects.

❊ Take a tincture of equal amounts of oats and vervain three times a day to nourish the nerves.

Headache

The causes of headaches are many and varied, but the most common are tension, dehydration, caffeine withdrawal, hormonal changes (see Menopause, page 24, and Premenstrual tension, page 247), high blood pressure (see page 230), eye strain, sinus congestion (see Sinusitis, page 225), infection (see page 237), dental problems and liver insufficiency. (See also Migraine, page 235.) The symptoms are a variety of different head pains ranging from throbbing to shooting pains. The location also varies from an isolated area to all over the whole head. Less commonly, they are caused by temporal arteritis, stroke, brain tumour and haemorrhage. Herbal treatment relies on identifying the cause and use of appropriate remedies.

Healing herbs
Mistletoe (see page 59)
Valerian (see page 79)
Chamomile (see page 102)
Wood betony (see page 111)
Cramp bark (see page 187)
Mint (see page 198)

Treatments

❊ Mistletoe is good for nerve pain, so take a tea or tincture of mistletoe for neuralgic headaches.

❊ Take a tea or tinctures of equal parts of valerian, wood betony and cramp bark for tension headaches. Take 10 ml (2 teaspoons) of the tincture every two hours.

❊ Take a strong infusion of mint and chamomile tea for headaches caused by digestive upset.

Insomnia

An inability to sleep. You may not be able to get off to sleep, or may wake during the night and not be able to go back to sleep. Early-morning waking is a feature of depression. Causes are stress, anxiety, altered sleep patterns from shift work or jetlag, low blood-sugar levels and excess caffeine. Central nervous system and sedative herbs will help to settle an over-active mind and promote a restful night's sleep. Nervous restorative remedies will aid healing of a depleted system.

Healing herbs
Lime (see page 56)
Valerian (see page 79)
Oat (see page 93)
Chamomile (see page 102)
Mugwort (see page 128)
Vervain (see page 161)
Hop (see page 178)

Treatments

❊ Take up to 15 ml ($1/2$ fl oz) valerian tincture in a little water before bed.

❊ Drink chamomile tea throughout the evening after a stressful day, to wind down.

❊ Take a tincture mix of equal parts St John's wort,

vervain and oat three times a day if suffering from prolonged stress or anxiety.

❋ Drink mugwort tea for its reputation to induce dreaming as dreams are our mind's way of processing problems.

❋ Drink limeflower tea as a pleasant relaxing tea.

❋ Add hop for its soporific effects.

Migraine

Debilitating recurrent headache, characterized by throbbing pains, that may be on one or both sides of the head, and may cause vomiting, visual disturbance and speech difficulties. It results from constriction and then dilation and engorgement of the blood vessels in the brain. Risk factors include red wine, cheese, chocolate, caffeine, hormone changes and stress. Stress migraines typically occur on the days off work.

Healing herbs

Mistletoe (see page 59)
Valerian (see page 79)
Wood betony (see page 111)
Mint (see page 198)
Feverfew (see page 201)

Treatments

❋ Take a fresh leaf of feverfew every day as a migraine preventative.

❋ Taking a tincture mix of equal parts wood betony and feverfew twice a day for a few months may help to reduce attacks.

❋ Take 15 ml ($1/2$ fl oz) tincture mix of equal parts mistletoe, valerian, feverfew and wood betony at the first sign of an attack. Repeat after an hour if required.

❋ Sip strong mint tea to alleviate nausea and support the liver.

Neuralgia

Neuralgia is nerve pain caused by damage from trauma, infections like shingles and various diseases like Multiple Sclerosis or diabetes. It can affect nerves anywhere in the body and the pain may be constant or intermittent. The symptoms vary from person to person. Herbal treatment will look to address the causative factors and to apply nervous system restoratives.

Healing herbs

Oat (see page 93)
St John's wort (see page 137)

Treatments

❋ Take a tincture or tea of St John's wort regularly to encourage nerve repair and restore function.

❋ Apply the infused oil of St John's wort regularly to the affected area for its pain-relieving effects.

❋ Take oats as food or as a tincture regularly to feed the nerves and provide them with the nourishment they require for healing.

The immune system

Allergies

Allergies are caused by the immune system over-reacting to the presence of foreign substances such as pollens, dust mites and animal dander. The symptoms can manifest as sneezing, streaming nose, itching of the eyes, nose, throat and skin, diarrhoea, and in severe situations swelling. This is in response to histamine produced by the body, which causes congestion in the tissues. The severe allergic reaction known as anaphylaxis requires urgent medical attention. If in doubt, call the emergency services.

Healing herbs
Chamomile (see page 102)
Plantain (see page 105)
Nettle (see page 155)
Elderflower (see page 184)
Milk thistle (see page 195)

Treatments
❋ Take equal parts nettle, chamomile and elderflower as a tea three times a day for antihistamine and mucous membrane tonic effects.
❋ Take 1 teaspoon ground milk thistle seeds on food twice a day to support the liver.
❋ Take plantain juice or tincture to cleanse the blood and boost the immune system.

Fever

A rise in body temperature in response to invading organisms and as a result of toxins released by those organisms. It is a sign that the body is fighting infection. It should not be suppressed, but supported and controlled using appropriate herbal remedies to induce natural cooling through sweating, which will also eliminate toxins. Normal body temperature is 36.9°C (98.6°F); a fever is considered to be anything above 37.2°C (99°F). Temperatures of 40°C (104°F) or above are dangerous. As a safe rule, if the temperature goes above 39.5°C (103°F), seek professional medical help and use paracetamol and tepid bathing to cool the body.

Healing herbs
Lime (see page 56)
Willow (see page 73)
Yarrow (see page 84)
Chamomile (see page 102)
Mugwort (see page 128)
Dog rose (see page 143)
Elderflower (see page 184)
Mint (see page 198)
Feverfew (see page 201)

Treatments
❋ Give children infusions of equal amounts of chamomile, limeflower and elderflower tea to drink freely, to open the pores and encourage sweating and encourage restful sleep.
❋ Babies of 3–6 months may be given a tepid bath with an infusion of these herb.
❋ For adults, drink a hot infusion of any combination

of the above herbs in equal amounts to promote sweating and encourage natural cooling.

Fungal infections

Most common fungal problems on the skin, such as athlete's foot and ringworm, are caused by tinea infections. They cause itching, redness, peeling skin and in ringworm a typical red ring. Candida fungal infections cause thrush and tend to affect the mucous membranes of the vagina and mouth, but may also affect the whole digestive tract in people with poor immune function. Vaginal thrush causes itching and a creamy, curd-like discharge from the vagina. In the mouth, white plaques with red sore areas are visible on the insides of the cheeks, the gums and the tongue.

Healing herbs
Wild garlic (see page 41)
Wood avens (see page 44)
Wild thyme (see page 204)

Treatments
❋ Eat wild garlic for its antifungal effects and to boost the immune system.
❋ Use the infused oil of wild garlic bulbs topically on the skin three times a day.
❋ Make an infusion of equal parts wood avens and wild thyme and use as a mouthwash for oral thrush, or as a douche for vaginal thrush. Do this three times a day.

Infection

The invasion of foreign organisms into the cells of the body. The body produces an immune response and the invading organisms often produce toxins that create varying symptoms depending on the source of infection. They may include fever, malaise, headaches, muscle aches and diarrhoea. Viruses, bacteria, funguses and parasites can all infect the body. (See also Fever, page 236; Cystitis, page 244; Sore throat, page 226; Bronchitis, page 222.)

Healing herbs
Wild garlic (see page 41)
Elderberry (see page 184)
Wild thyme (see page 204)

Treatments
❋ For viral infections, take elderberry tincture or compound every two hours for eight doses, then four times a day until better.
❋ Eat wild garlic leaves and bulbs for a powerful anti-infective effect.
❋ Drink wild thyme tea every four hours for bacterial infections and three times a day for fungal infections.

The digestive system

Bloating

An uncomfortable condition of the digestive system, creating feelings of fullness and a distended abdomen. It may be a feature of irritable bowel syndrome (see page 242). It may be caused by insufficient digestive enzymes resulting in sluggish passage of food through the digestive tract and fermentation of food, and the presence of unbalanced gut bacteria. Many women notice it at different times of their menstrual cycle and it can be due to an over-loaded liver and the digestion being affected by hormones. Treatment with herbs aims to provide wind dispersive and anti-spasmodic effects, improve liver and digestive function and rebalance gut bacteria.

Healing herbs
Dandelion root (see page 114)
Milk thistle (see page 195)
Mint (see page 198)
Wild thyme (see page 204)

Treatments
❋ Drink mint tea up to three times a day after meals to regulate contraction of the gut and reduce spasm (avoid in heartburn).
❋ Take dandelion root as a tincture up to three times a day to support the liver and improve digestion.
❋ Use thyme in food, as an infusion or as a tincture up to three times a day if gut flora are imbalanced.
❋ Take milk thistle tincture twice a day to improve liver function.

Colic

A painful spasm of the intestines and bowel, probably caused by wind and tension. It is usually seen in babies, but adults may also suffer from it. Babies cry or scream for long periods, draw up their legs to their tummies and pass wind. There are many theories as to the causes, including aggravation by foods ingested by breastfeeding mothers (spices, brassicas, sugar, dairy products, etc) and immature intestines developing gut bacteria that cause wind. In adults, it may also be caused by food sensitivities, irritable bowel syndrome (see page 242) or by the passage of or blockage by a gallstone or kidney stone (see Gallstones, page 241; Kidney stones, page 244). Antispasmodic herbs relax tense, painful muscle spasms via the central nervous system, and directly on the nerve endings in the intestines. Carminative herbs help to disperse wind.

Healing herbs
Valerian (see page 79)
Chamomile (see page 102)
Hop (see page 178)
Cramp bark (see page 187)
Mint (see page 198)
Wild thyme (see page 204)

Treatments
❋ Breastfeeding mothers can drink chamomile tea up to four times a day to help them relax; its antispasmodic effects will pass to the baby through the breast milk.

❋ Gently massage infused oil of chamomile into the baby's tummy and feet.

❋ Bathe the baby with infusion of chamomile in the water. They will absorb it into their system through the skin.

❋ For adults, make a tincture mix of equal parts valerian, hop, mint and cramp bark and take 20 ml (3/4 fl oz) in sips from a glass of water.

❋ Sip an infusion of wild thyme tea to disperse wind and reduce spasm.

Constipation

Difficulty in opening bowels regularly and difficult elimination of hard, dry faeces may be caused by too high or too low a bowel tone, low dietary fibre and fluid intake, and poor liver function. It is commonly experienced during pregnancy, while travelling, and by the elderly. Bitter liver herbs stimulate efficient digestion and improve and ease bowel movements.

Healing herbs
Fumitory (see page 99)
Plantain (see page 105)
Yellow dock (see page 108)
Dandelion (see page 114)
Burdock (see page 125)
Vervain (see page 161)
Elderberry (see page 184)
Sweet violet (see page 207)

Treatments
❋ Take 1–2 teaspoons violet flower syrup as a gentle laxative for children.

❋ Take a combination of 1 part yellow dock or fumitory, 2 parts burdock and 2 parts dandelion root tincture three times a day to improve liver function and improve bowel function.

❋ For constipation caused by anxiety and tension, take vervain tea up to three times a day, or 10 ml (2 teaspoons) tincture twice a day.

❋ Take up to 1 dessertspoon plantain seeds on food for their bulking, laxative effects.

❋ Eat raw or cooked elderberries for their laxative effects. Beware as they can be potent!

Diarrhoea

The symptoms are abdominal cramps and the passing of frequent, watery stools that may be explosive and urgent. It may be caused by infection by a virus or bacterium, inflammatory disease such as Crohn's disease and ulcerative colitis, irritable bowel syndrome (see page 242), parasite or coeliac disease. Infections may be caused by contaminated food, contact with contaminated surfaces or acute diverticulitis (see page 240) and should resolve within a week. Diarrhoea that continues longer than a week requires investigation. A complication of diarrhoea is dehydration, especially in children and the elderly. Prolonged changes in bowel habit should be investigated. Inflammatory bowel disease is very complex and requires expert treatment with a trained medical herbalist; however, soothing astringent herbal teas are beneficial if taken daily to tone up the mucous membranes and reduce inflammation.

Healing herbs
Wood avens (see page 44)
Oak (see page 47)
Mallow (see page 64)
Silverweed (see page 70)
Agrimony (see page 87)
Chamomile (see page 102)

The digestive system

Plantain (see page 105)
Shepherd's purse (see page 131)
Dog rose (see page 143)
White deadnettle (see page 181)
Mint (see page 198)

Treatments

❋ Drink teas of any combination of the above herbs in equal parts to remain hydrated, and for their soothing, tonic effects on the bowel.
❋ Take oak bark tincture twice a day for a powerful astringent action.
❋ Drink equal parts plantain, chamomile and agrimony as a tea three times a day to tone and soothe the bowel.

Diverticular disease

A condition caused by small pockets of the large bowel becoming chronically enlarged. The risk factors of this developing are chronic constipation, low dietary fibre intake and ageing. They may become periodically impacted with faeces, causing infection and inflammation known as diverticulitis. Symptoms of diverticulitis are pain, diarrhoea and general malaise. Complications may be perforation and bleeding of the bowel.

Healing herbs

Wild garlic (see page 41)
Agrimony (see page 87)
Plantain (see page 105)
Yellow dock (see page 108)
Hop (see page 178)
Cramp bark (see page 187)
Mint (see page 198)
Wild thyme (see page 204)

Treatments

❋ To tone the bowel, drink equal parts agrimony and plantain tea up to three times a day.
❋ For constipation, take yellow dock tincture 2–3 times a day.
❋ Take up to 1 dessertspoon plantain seeds, on food, every day for constipation.
❋ For acute infection, eat the leaves or bulb of wild garlic every four hours.
❋ For infection, take wild thyme tea every four hours for its antiseptic properties.
❋ For pain and spasm, drink mint tea up to six times a day, or take 5 ml (1 teaspoon) of a mix of equal amounts of hops and cramp bark tincture every four hours.

Flatulence

Belching or passing wind from the bowels. Causes of belching are eating too fast and gulping down poorly chewed food, thus swallowing lots of air. It is also a sign of insufficient stomach acid and slow gastric emptying, causing food to ferment in the stomach and gas to be formed. Wind from the bowel is caused by gas passing through from the stomach, and from fermentation and gas formation by bacteria during the digestive process. Some foods increase flatulence, such as brassicas and pulses.

Healing herbs

Chamomile (see page 102)
Dandelion root (see page 114)
Horseradish (see page 122)
Mint (see page 198)
Wild thyme (see page 204)

Treatments

❋ Include horseradish in the diet to increase stomach acid and improve digestion.

❋ Drink an infusion of equal parts thyme, mint and chamomile after meals for their carminative effects.

❋ Drink dandelion coffee (see page 116) before meals to stimulate the production of digestive enzymes.

Gallstones

Stones form in the bile duct, due to precipitation of cholesterol and bile pigments out of the bile. Traditional risk factors include the 'five Fs' – fair, female, fertile, fat and forty – although this is not strictly true, as men also frequently suffer with them. They can cause acute pain under the ribs on the right-hand side and indigestion. They are aggravated by fatty foods and may be complicated by a stone becoming lodged in the bile duct causing obstructive jaundice and biliary colic. Herbal protocols aim to thin and increase production of the bile to reduce production of more stones and keep the bile moving.

Healing herbs

Agrimony (see page 87)
Fumitory (see page 99)
Dandelion root (see page 114)
Hop (see page 178)
Cramp bark (see page 187)
Milk thistle (see page 195)

Treatments

❋ Drink dandelion coffee (see page 116) up to three times a day to stimulate flow of bile.

❋ Drink agrimony tea as a simple to improve liver function and bowel health.

❋ Take a tincture mix of equal parts of fumitory, milk thistle and dandelion root up to three times a day to stimulate bile production.

❋ Take equal parts of fumitory, cramp bark and hop tincture every two hours to relieve the pain of an attack of biliary colic.

Hangover

This occurs as a consequence of excessive consumption of alcohol. Symptoms are headache, nausea, sensitivity to light and sound, thirst, fatigue and dizziness. The alcohol acts like a poison on the system and causes dehydration, blood-sugar imbalances, sleep disturbance and nervous system effects. Symptoms resolve with time as the liver slowly metabolizes the alcohol and toxins are eliminated. The more alcohol drunk, the longer the recovery.

Healing herbs

Chamomile (see page 102)
Plantain (see page 105)
Milk thistle (see page 195)

Treatments

❋ Take milk thistle tincture before and after drinking alcohol to protect the cells of the liver from the damaging effects of alcohol.

❋ Take equal parts of chamomile and plantain tea to relieve the symptoms of nausea and headache, and to rehydrate the body.

❋ Add wood betony if headache is present.

Heartburn

Reflux of stomach acid up into the oesophagus gives a sensation of burning and discomfort in the centre of the chest. It may even extend as far as the back of the throat, leading to a bitter taste in the mouth. Causes are hiatus hernia (a weakness and bulge of the stomach through the diaphragm) and over- or under-production of acid in the stomach (for under-production, see Indigestion, below). Over-production is usually a result of stress and anxiety.

Healing herbs
Mallow root (see page 64)
Comfrey (see page 76)
Chamomile (see page 102)
Plantain (see page 105)
Meadowsweet (see page 169)

Treatments
❊ Take a tea or tinctures of any of the above herbs in equal parts, three times a day, to soothe the membranes of the oesophagus and tone the sphincter between it and the stomach.

Indigestion
Indigestion is an uncomfortable feeling of fullness and acidity in the stomach, often after consuming food. Causes are over-eating, insufficient digestive acid and food sensitivities. Acidity that occurs on an empty stomach is caused by an inflamed stomach lining, which can be triggered by stress, gallstones and non-steroidal anti-inflammatory drugs such as aspirin.

Healing herbs
Mallow (see page 64)
Chamomile (see page 102)
Plantain (see page 105)
Dandelion (see page 114)
Horseradish (see page 122)
Mugwort (see page 128)

Elecampane (see page 140)
Meadowsweet (see page 169)
Ground ivy (see page 175)
Milk thistle (see page 195)

Treatments
❊ For acidity when the stomach is empty, take equal parts of mallow, chamomile, plantain and meadowsweet tea for their anti-inflammatory effects.
❊ For indigestion after food, take 1–2 teaspoons horseradish composition (see page 123) before food.
❊ Take milk thistle and dandelion tincture 20 minutes before meals to improve digestion.
❊ Take dandelion coffee (see page 116) to improve liver function and digestion.

Irritable bowel syndrome (IBS)
This condition is a disorder of the system that controls mobility of the bowel. The core symptoms are recurrent abdominal pain, often with changes in bowel habit from constipation to diarrhoea. Studies have shown that one in three cases of IBS results from the sufferer having some kind of food allergy or intolerance and poor digestion. Stress and depression are also contributing factors. Herbal treatment depends on identifying individual causes.

Healing herbs
Wood avens (see page 44)
Siverweed (see page 70)
Valerian (see page 79)
Agrimony (see page 87)
Chamomile (see page 102)
Wood betony (see page 111)
Dandelion (see page 114)
Hop (see page 178)

Cramp bark (see page 187)
Mint (see page 198)

Treatments

❋ Take a tea or standard-dose tincture of chamomile 3–6 times a day.

❋ To improve digestion, take dandelion coffee (see page 116) as a substitute for regular coffee, which is a bowel irritant.

❋ Use a tincture of equal parts of any of mint, hop, cramp bark and valerian for pain and spasm.

❋ Use silverweed or agrimony as a tea or tincture if diarrhoea is a problem.

Nausea

Feeling sick may be caused by infection, pregnancy, headaches and liver disease. In stomach bugs or food poisoning, it may precede vomiting, so do not eat or drink anything for a few hours until the nausea stops, rinsing the mouth with water if required. Do not eat until feelings of hunger return, and sip fluids slowly.

Healing herbs

Chamomile (see page 102)
Dandelion (see page 114)
Mint (see page 198)

Treatments

❋ Sip a cup of chamomile tea for nausea and after vomiting, when reintroducing fluids (suitable for use during pregnancy).

❋ For morning sickness, drink dandelion coffee (see page 116) to support the liver.

❋ Sip peppermint tea for nausea from liverishness or over-eating (take with caution during pregnancy).

Worms

Pin or thread worms are the most common worm infestation seen in children. They cause itching of the anus at night as the female worms come out to lay eggs. The eggs are then introduced into the digestive tract by hand to mouth, where they are swallowed. They then hatch in the intestines and the process begins again. Hygiene is essential to prevent reinfection. Washing hands, wearing pants in bed and washing bed linen and clothes on a hot wash regularly will help prevent reinfection. The worms thrive on sugar consumed in the diet. Eating grated carrots and pumpkin seeds every day, on an empty stomach, will help to kill the worms in the intestine.

Healing herbs

Wild garlic (see page 41)
Dandelion (see page 114)
Mugwort (see page 128)

Treatments

❋ Eat a raw wild garlic bulb three times a day for ten days. It is important to smell of garlic as it is the volatile oil that kills them.

❋ Drink dandelion coffee (see page 116) every day to increase bile flow.

The urinary system

Cystitis

Cystitis is an uncomfortable infection of the bladder and urinary tract that can also be caused by bruising to the urethra. It can be a recurrent or chronic condition. Bacteria spread from the anus from wearing tight trousers, wiping back to front after defecation, or as a result of sexual intercourse during which the urethra may be bruised (this is why it is also known as 'honeymooners' disease'). Symptoms are painful, burning and frequent urination. The urine may smell offensive and be tinged pink by blood. Women are more prone than men, as the female urethra is shorter than the male urethra which means that infective bacteria may migrate up into the bladder more easily.

Healing herbs

Mallow (see page 64)
Horsetail (see page 67)
Silverweed (see page 70)
Yarrow (see page 84)
Couch grass (see page 90)
Plantain (see page 105)
Dandelion (see page 114)
Shepherd's purse (see page 131)
Golden rod (see page 146)
Chickweed (see page 149)
Cleavers (see page 172)
Ground ivy (see page 175)
Elder (see page 184)
Wild thyme (see page 204)

Treatments

❋ Take copious amounts of warm teas of any combinations of the above herbs to increase urination and flush the bacteria out. Mallow and couch grass are soothing demulcents; thyme, golden rod and ground ivy are antibacterial; yarrow and golden rod are diuretic; and plantain is antibacterial and soothing.

Incontinence

Incontinence has a number of different causes including: damage to the nerves supplying the bladder either from disease, trauma or recurrent infection, acute infection, damage to the supporting muscles and ligaments of the bladder usually from pregnancy and childbirth, prostate enlargement (see prostate problems) and childhood enuresis (bedwetting). Herbal regimes depend largely on the cause. (See also Cystitis and Prostate problems.)

Healing Herbs

Horsetail (see page 67)
Plantain (see page 105)
Shepherds purse (see page 131)
St John's wort (see page 137)

Treatments

❋ Take shepherd's purse tea or tincture regularly to improve the tone of the ligaments surrounding the bladder especially if stress incontinence is a problem from childbirth.

❋ Horsetail juice tea or tincture has a restorative

effect on all of the tissues of the bladder due to its silica content.

❋ St John's wort tea or tincture is indicated if nerve irritation or damage is a problem, to restore function.

❋ Plantain tea or tincture taken long term is useful for the symptoms of chronic cystitis.

Kidney stones

These are most commonly formed by excess calcium in the urinary system. Kidney stones may pass from the kidney to the bladder, via the urethra, causing the excruciating pain of renal colic. Risk factors include antacid medication, chronic dehydration and thyroid disease. Increased fluid intake is essential to prevent the formation of further stones.

Healing herbs
Mallow (see page 64)
Horsetail (see page 67)
Couch grass (see page 90)
Dandelion leaf (see page 114)
Golden rod (see page 146)
Cleavers (see page 172)
Ground ivy (see page 175)
Cramp bark (see page 187)

Treatments
❋ For renal colic, drink a warm tea of equal amounts of any of the following: couch grass, cleavers, ground ivy, dandelion, golden rod and mallow every two hours to increase urine flow and soothe any irritation.

❋ If the urine is bloodstained, take a tea of mallow and horsetail to prevent bleeding.

❋ Take 5 ml (1 teaspoon) cramp bark tincture every two hours for pain.

Prostate problems

Symptoms are caused by enlargement of the prostate gland in men; this condition is most commonly benign, but may be caused by malignancy. The symptoms are frequency, urgency and poor flow of urine during the day and at night. It is often seen as a consequence of ageing in men. Infection may be a problem if urine is being retained in the bladder (see Cystitis, page 244).

Healing herbs
Horsetail (see page 67)
Couch grass (see page 90)
Plantain (see page 105)
Nettle root (see page 155)

Treatments
❋ Take a tincture mix of horsetail and nettle root three times a day as a genito-urinary tonic.

❋ For blood in the urine, take a tea of plantain, horsetail and couch grass. Drink freely to increase urine flow and soothe membranes.

The urinary system

The reproductive system

Menopause

The cessation of menstruation and fertility is a natural part of the female ageing process, and commonly occurs anywhere between 45 and 60 years of age. Menstrual disturbance as a result of the reduction of oestrogen in the body may be the first sign. Other symptoms include hot flushes, night sweats, mood swings, inability to concentrate and poor memory. The whole process varies for each individual as the body adapts. Symptoms respond well to herbal and dietary regimes that provide gentle-acting, plant-based, hormone-like effects and assist the body in adapting to the change in hormone levels without the regular cycle of reproductive hormones.

Healing herbs

Oat (see page 93)
Dandelion root (see page 114)
Red clover (see page 117)
St John's wort (see page 137)
Vervain (see page 161)
Hop (see page 178)

Treatments

❋ Take a tea or tincture of hop and red clover for their oestrogen-like properties. Hops are specific for night sweats. Add St John's wort and vervain for anxiety and mood swings.
❋ Take dandelion coffee (see page 116) daily to support the liver and its metabolism of hormones.
❋ Take oats in the diet or as a tincture to support the nervous system if anxiety is a problem.

Periods, heavy

It is difficult to measure what constitutes a heavy period, as this varies from person to person. The average menstrual blood loss per period is said to be around 75 ml (3 fl oz). Bleeding more than this, or regularly lasting for 8–10 days, is also considered to be heavy. The presence of large clots is indicative of pelvic blood flow congestion, and is seen in teenage women, as periods establish themselves, and in menopause. It is associated with fibroids, endometriosis, uterine polyps, pelvic inflammatory disease and dysfunctional uterine bleeding, which is poorly understood.

Healing herbs

Silverweed (see page 70)
Yarrow (see page 84)
Shepherd's purse (see page 131)
Dog rose (see page 143)
Nettle (see page 155)
White deadnettle (see page 181)

Treatments

❋ Drink nettle tea three times a day for its astringent properties and iron-rich content.
❋ Make a tincture mix of equal parts of any of the following: White deadnettle, dog rose petals, silverweed and shepherd's purse, and take three times a day for at least three cycles, for their astringent properties.

❋ If pain precedes bleeding and then clots are present, take yarrow as a tea or tincture three times a day to promote pelvic blood flow. They are also beneficial for their astringent properties to tone up the uterine blood vessels.

Periods, painful

If the pain starts before the bleeding, and is a dull ache and 'dragging' in sensation, and eases off as the flow becomes established, it is congestive dysmenorrhoea and is due to sluggish pelvic blood flow. This occurs more frequently in older women. If the pain is cramping and spasmodic, and starts as flow becomes established, it is spasmodic dysmenorrhoea and is caused by inflammatory prostaglandin chemicals. This is usually experienced by younger women.

Healing herbs
Valerian (see page 79)
Yarrow (see page 84)
Chamomile (see page 105)
Mugwort (see page 128)
Cramp bark (see page 187)
Feverfew (see page 201)

Treatments
❋ For congestive pain, make a tea of 3 parts yarrow and 1 part mugwort. Drink this tea twice a day in the week leading up to menstruation to improve pelvic blood flow.
❋ For spasmodic pain, make a mix of equal parts of valerian, cramp bark and feverfew tinctures and take 10 ml (2 teaspoons) every two hours at the start of the period for their antispasmodic and anti-inflammatory effects.

Premenstrual tension (PMT)

Various symptoms are experienced by women in the weeks leading up to the start of their period, including mood swings, water retention, breast tenderness, sugar cravings, headaches and lower abdominal or back pain. PMT is probably caused by sensitivity to hormone changes leading up to menstruation. Symptoms resolve once the period has started. Stress, caffeine intake, alcohol and a poor diet that is high in refined carbohydrates may aggravate the condition.

Healing herbs
Oat (see page 93)
Dandelion root (see page 114)
St John's wort (see page 137)
Vervain (see page 161)
Milk thistle (see page 195)

Treatments
❋ Drink dandelion coffee (see page 116) or milk thistle tincture or ground seed to improve liver metabolism of hormones.
❋ If stress and anxiety are present, take a tincture mix of equal parts vervain, St John's wort and oat three times a day to feed and support the nerves.

First aid kit – top ten healing plants

These are the ten herbs that have the most versatile and wide-ranging properties and can be used to treat most common ailments. Try to gather and prepare enough to last all year until the next growing season and harvesting time.

HERB	GOOD FOR	PREPARATIONS
Chamomile (see page 102)	Allergies, anxiety and stress, insomnia, fever, nausea, irritable bowel syndrome (IBS), indigestion, colic, heartburn, gastritis, eczema	Dried herb, infused oil, fresh herb tincture
Nettle (see page 155)	Allergies, arthritis, osteoporosis, gout, iron deficiency, bleeding, end stage of pregnancy and after labour, falling hair, dandruff, adrenal restorative, prostate problems	Dried herb, fresh herb tincture, dried nettle seed, root tincture
Elder (see page 184	Fever, colds, catarrh, hayfever, allergies, dry skin, bacterial and viral infections, flu	Dried flowers, fresh flower tincture, infused flower oil, dried berries, berry syrup, fresh berry tincture
Wild thyme (see page 204)	Coughs, bloating, flatulence, infections, sore throat, fungal infections	Dried herb, fresh herb tincture, infused oil, syrup
Yarrow (see page 84)	Fever, colds, infections, cystitis, painful periods, high blood pressure, chilblains, circulation problems, haemorrhoids (piles), eczema	Dried herb, infused oil, fresh herb tincture

First aid kit

HERB	GOOD FOR	PREPARATIONS
Mint (see page 198)	Headache, nausea, flatulence, bloating, irritable bowel syndrome (IBS), catarrh, colds	Dried herb, fresh herb tincture
Plantain (see page 105)	Allergies, hayfever, psoriasis, eczema, indigestion, gastritis, heartburn, bleeding, haemorrhoids (piles), bites and stings, wounds	Dried herb, fresh herb tincture, infused oil
Oat (see page 93)	Exhaustion, anxiety and stress, depression, convalescence, cold sores, chickenpox and shingles, myalgic encephalitis (ME), chronic fatigue syndrome, dry skin	Fresh herb tincture
Dandelion (see page 114)	Indigestion, poor appetite, gallstones, irritable bowel syndrome (IBS), flatulence, bloating, constipation, acne, psoriasis, gout, arthritis, water retention, warts and verrucas	Dried root, fresh root tincture, fresh herb tincture, dandelion coffee
St John's wort (see page 137)	Anxiety and stress, insomnia, nerve damage and neuralgia, depression, cold sores, chickenpox and shingles, premenstrual tension (PMT), menopause, burns, psoriasis.	Dried herb, fresh herb tincture, infused oil

Glossary

Abortifacient
Substance that causes or promotes abortion.

Adaptogen
Substance that increases the body's ability to adapt to internal or external stress.

Alterative
Gradually alters or changes a condition by improving the body's function.

Analgesic
Relieves pain and discomfort.

Annual plant
A plant that completes its life cycle (grows and sets seed) in one year.

Antacid
Neutralizes stomach acid.

Antibiotic
Kills or inhibits the growth of bacteria and other micro–organisms.

Anticoagulant
Reduces clotting ability of the blood.

Antidepressant
Helps to lift low mood.

Antihelminic
Destroys and expels worms. Also called vermifuge.

Anti–inflammatory
Reduces heat, redness and swelling.

Antiseptic
Destroys bacteria; usually applied externally.

Antispasmodic
Relieves or prevents muscle spasms or cramps.

Antitussive
Stops a cough.

Aromatic
Has a strong odour, usually due to its volatile oils.

Astringent
Tightens up relaxed tissues. Used to stop bleeding and excess discharges, and to close pores.

Biennial plant
A plant that completes its life cycle (grows and sets seed) in two years.

Bitter tonic
A bitter taste that stimulates the flow of gastric juices.

Calmative
Has a calming effect; usually not as strong as a sedative.

Carminative
Dispels or prevents gas.

Cholagogue
Promotes the flow of bile.

Decongestant
Reduces congestion in the upper respiratory tract.

Demulcent
Mucilaginous substance that soothes and moistens irritated tissues.

Diaphoretic
Promotes sweating.

Diuretic
Promotes the flow of urine.

Doctrine of Signatures
The belief that God gave each medicinal plant a sign to indicate what it was good for. For example, the orange sap of celandine for bile.

Emetic
Induces vomiting.

Emmenagogue
Promotes menstruation.

Emollient
Softens and soothes the skin.

Expectorant
Expels phlegm by stimulating the respiratory tract.

Febrifuge
Reduces a fever.

Flatulence
Gas in the stomach or bowels.

Galactagogue
Increases breast milk production.

Hemostatic
Stops blood flow.

Hepatic
Has an effect on the liver.

Herbal
A book about herbs or plants, describing their kinds, qualities, uses and so on.

Laxative
Has an action on the bowel, stimulating a bowel movement.

Nervine
Calms nervousness, tension and excitement.

Perennial plant
A plant that dies down and then re-grows year after year.

Purgative
A strong cathartic, irritating the bowel wall.

Refrigerant
Cools the blood and reduces fever.

Rubefacient
Increases blood circulation to an area where it is applied, reddening the skin.

Sedative
Reduces nervous tension and induces relaxation.

Simple
A herb used individually for treatment.

Soporific
Induces sleep.

Stimulant
Increases or quickens actions of the body.

Styptic
Stops external bleeding.

Topical
Used externally, applied to the skin.

Tonic
Strengthens and invigorates a system.

Vermifuge
See Antihelminic.

Vulnerary
Used to treat wounds.

Resources

TO FIND A MEDICAL HERBALIST
The National Institute of Medical Herbalists
www.nimh.org
The College of Practitioners of Phytotherapy
www.cpp.co.uk

USEFUL RESOURCES
A Modern Herbal by Mrs M Grieve
The Concise British Floral in Colour by W. Keeble Martin 1969
The British Herbal Pharmacopea 1983
Henriettes Herbal Website www.henriettesherbal.com

SUPPLIERS of herbs, jars, bottles and sundries
Neals Yard Remedies www.nealsyardremedies.com
Baldwins www.baldwins.co.uk
Proline Botanicals www.prolinebotanicals.com
The Organic Herb Trading Company
www.organicherbtrading.com

HONEY AND BEESWAX
To find your local beekeeper who may sell his produce, visit:
www.britishbee.org.uk

Index

Acknowledgements

Thank you to fellow Medical Herbalists: Margaret Macmillan for her attention to detail, Sue Hawkey for wise words of support, Max Drake for a shared passion of becoming a self sustainable herbalist and Anne Brennan for a generous listening ear. Thanks to my friends and family for being trusting and willing guinea pigs. Finally thank you to Kerenza and Jessica for their patience and belief in me.

Executive Editor Jessica Cowie
Editor Kerenza Swift
Executive Art Editor Leigh Jones
Designer Janis Utton
Production Controller David Hearn

All photographs are by Zoë Hawes with the exception of the following:
Alamy Andrew Darrington 182, Arco Images GmbH 56, 206, blickwinkel 48, 146, 176, David Chapman 147, 174, LOOK Die Bildagentur der Fotografen GmbH 50, Marie-Louise Avery 9, Martin Fowler 98, Nigel Cattlin 92, Organics Image Library 71, Photofrenetic 44, 159, Zeno Elea 75
BotanikFoto Steffen Hauser 77, 203
Dreamstime.com Arfo 199
Fotolia Dmitry Argunov 152, Karen Popovich 195, photlook 60
Getty Images Michael Melford 47
istockphoto.com Douglas Atmore 197, Juanmonino 32, Liudmila Otrutskaya 168, Nancy Nehring 160, Predrag Novakovic 194, Roger Whiteway 158, 185, Ruud de Man 166
Photolibrary Elliott Neep 67, J S Sira 81, Mark Bolton 190, Torbjorn Arvidson 154, Ute Klaphake 106
Photoshot NHPA/Laurie Campbell 99, Stephen Dalton 194
S & O Mathews Oliver Mathews 100
Shutterstock Adrian Grosu 136, Aleksander Bolbot 36, Alex Kosev 144, Alexey Andreevich Kuznetsov 13, David Maska 180
Stockfood Food Photography Eising 34